RAPID WEIGHT LOSS HYPNOSIS FOR WOMEN:

The Ultimate Guide To Hypnosis, Meditation, And Affirmations For Rapid Weight Loss. How To Get Lean By Increasing Motivation And Controlling Emotional Eating.

NORMA JOHNSON

Table Of Contents

4

Introduction

Hypnosis is the technique that allows you to go into that state of your consciousness wherein you allow the part of your brain in charge of your subconscious to dominate your thought process. That means that when you are being hypnotized, you tap the right hemisphere of your brain, which is in charge of your automatic actions, creativity, and imagination.

Hypnosis also makes you very susceptible to suggestions and influence, and since you are suppressing the part of your brain that dictates logic, you are able to suspend your current beliefs about what you can do. That allows this technique to make suggestions, make your mind allow suppressed memories to resurface, or even help you change your own behavior.

Hypnosis has been a very controversial technique – because it can make a person think of things that he would usually would not, to the point that it can lead a person to perform things that appear to be outside his will, some view this technique to be dangerous.

However, a deeper understanding of what happens during hypnosis will make you really see what may happen under a hypnotic trance and up to what point can a person really be commanded under hypnosis. In the end, you would also have a better understanding of how a person's mind can be manipulated.

What Happens When You are Hypnotized?

Whenever you enter a hypnotic trance, you would describe the feeling to be very similar to what you experience when you are daydreaming. You can imagine things that you usually cannot, the same as what your mind triggers while you are in the state of a dream when sleeping. You can imagine yourself flying, doing the real Superman punch, and so on, but the thing is, you are awake and hyper-attentive.

Why do people think that when you are hypnotized, you are actually in a sleep state? The reason is that when you are focusing intensely on anything that you want to indeed pay attention to, you lose yourself. It is similar to watching a movie or reading a book – you feel that all scenarios may happen in real life, and your emotions are engaged.

You suspend your beliefs for a moment and then enjoy the possibilities that are presented to you. Similar to reading a book or watching a movie, it is up to you to believe if what you are watching or reading can really happen in real life. That means that you have complete free will to believe or do anything under hypnosis – you can choose whether you want to resist an order or a suggestion that is offered to you. If you choose not to participate with the hypnosis, then there is nothing that a hypnotist can do to make you do an action or think of a thought.

Why does this happen? Whenever you allow access to your subconscious in a hypnosis session, you may feel that you are in a state of relaxation, but you are truly awake. Because you are allowing yourself to surrender to your imagination, your subconscious begins to work behind the scenes and projects images and scenarios in your mind. However, your conscious mind is still actively participating in your thoughts, and you can still know that some of the things that you see would not be possible in real life. However, your subconscious would still allow you to make use of your emotions.

Once your emotions are triggered in the event that your subconscious projects inside your mind, you would be able to formulate ideas using your conscious mind. This makes you feel inspired or have a particular idea that you can execute while you are fully conscious.

CHAPTER 1:

Hypnosis

I n reality, it is sometimes difficult to distinguish what is scientifically proven and what is not. For example, we know that psychology can help us lose weight, but we don't know much about other somewhat more confusing methods, such as hypnosis.

Is it possible that hypnosis helps us lose weight? Next, we analyze how they use hypnotherapy in different clinics that offer it as a method to lose weight and what the scientific research says about it.

Myths of Hypnosis

There are too many mistakes regarding hypnosis, many of which have been broadcast by movies that deal with people turned into zombies by an extremely powerful person who exclaims: "Look me in the eye!" This may be interesting, but It is mere fiction and has no relation to the truth. Next, we will expose some of the most common myths and explain them.

A person who is hypnotized can do things against his will. Completely false. First, nobody can be hypnotized against their will. It is essential that the subject wishes to cooperate. Secondly, no person who has been hypnotized can be forced to do something they would not do in a normal state. During hypnosis, the subject can accept or reject any suggested order. If what the hypnotist proposes disturbs the subject, in all likelihood he will quickly leave the hypnotic state.

It is only possible to hypnotize people with weak minds. The opposite is true. The smarter a person is, the easier it will be to hypnotize him. In fact, in certain cases of mental weakness it is absolutely impossible to practice hypnosis. It is possible to hypnotize practically all those who wish to be hypnotized. Only 1 percent of the population cannot be hypnotized due to mental deficiencies or other reasons beyond our understanding.

A hypnotized person is in a trance or unconscious. Absolutely fake. A subject undergoing hypnosis is awake and aware: extremely conscious. What happens is that he has simply focused his attention where the hypnotist has indicated and has abstracted himself from everything else.

Anyone can remain in a hypnotic state forever. This is completely false. Even assuming that the hypnotist died after hypnotizing the subject, he would leave the hypnotic state easily, either falling into a short sleep and then waking normally or opening his eyes when he did not hear the hypnotist's voice for a while.

To obtain positive results, a state of deep hypnosis is necessary. Is not true. Any level of hypnosis can offer good results.

HYPNOTIC STATE. -

Any person undergoing hypnosis is very aware of where they are and what is happening. The subject hears everything that happens while immersed in a state similar to daytime sleep, deeply relaxed. He often feels the body numb or has no awareness of having a body.

SELF HYPNOSIS

It is possible to self-hypnotize. Many people do it daily to give constructive orders. It is much easier to self-hypnotize if you have already gone through the experience of having been hypnotized by another person and received the instructions to do so. Through this book you will learn to hypnotize other people but with the same instructions you will learn to self-hypnotize. If you work with someone who hypnotizes you, you will accelerate the spread of self-hypnosis learning.

How Hypnosis Works to Lose Weight

People who carry out hypnosis treatments to lose weight use different methods. The general idea is to create in the patient changes in the way he sees himself, provide him with a state of relaxation and encourage his taste for a healthy meal.

One of the techniques they use is the induction of Dave Elman, which consists in relaxing the patient and, later, making him imagine a staircase with a mirror on the wall along the entire staircase. In that mirror he has to visualize a positive image of himself - in this case a thin version of himself. As you go down the stairs, you must melt your image with the image of the mirror to record a new mental image of yourself.

In other cases, one of the hypnoband is made, a method used by some celebrities such as Caritina Goyanes, who claimed in an interview to have been a success , in which during hypnosis, through relaxation, the unconscious that carries a gastric band is led to believe , although the patient knows that he is not wearing it.

Another method used is the post-hypnotic suggestions: instructions that are given to the subject once he is in the state of relaxation caused by hypnosis and that, presumably, would be recorded in his mind.

All these techniques can be found in a web browsing of clinics and centers that offer hypnotherapy as a method to help us lose weight.

JOAQUIN HEN

What science tells us about hypnosis for weight loss

The reality is that, from the year 2000 onwards, research has barely been carried out with respect to the effect that hypnosis could have as a weight loss treatment.

In 2014, a study was conducted on the etiology of obesity and the role that hypnosis could have in its identification and resolution. In their results they indicate that hypnotherapy could help modify the habits that maintain obesity. They themselves clarify that these results are found when hypnosis is used as a complement to an obesity treatment that includes changes in eating behavior and exercise.

The curious thing about this study is not only the results, but in the study itself they warn that the research carried out in this regard is minimal and outdated, so, despite having found allegedly positive results, the study authors themselves indicate that Hypnotherapy cannot ask to be taken seriously as a method of weight loss.

They are not wrong. This type of research began to be carried out approximately 30 years ago, but they are very scarce and contradictory.

One of the first was that carried out by Kirsch in 1995. They conducted a meta-analysis of 18 studies in which the effect on weight loss was compared between studies that only studied people who were taking a treatment based on cognitive therapy, and others in the that the same therapy was complemented with hypnotherapy.

In the results of the meta-analysis they found that, apparently, the weight loss could be greater when the two treatments were combined and that, in addition, those who had received a combined treatment, continued to lose weight after the treatment.

Hypnotize Me

In any case, the research authors themselves indicated that the correlation between hypnosis and weight loss results did not give information to explain the causative mechanism of hypnosis. That is, there was a correlation, but it was not explained by what mechanisms hypnosis could cause weight loss.

Later, in 1996, a new study was carried out, reviewing the results of the one carried out by Kirsch in 1995. In this new study, they found that Kirsch's meta-analysis had methodological errors. After controlling some of these errors, such as correcting some transcription and computational inaccuracies, they found that the effect of hypnosis, if any, was minimal.

Moreover, Allison and his team, authors of this new meta-analysis, find that by withdrawing one of the researchers studied in the original meta-analysis, considering it quite questionable, the effects were no longer statistically significant.

In 1998 a new study was carried out in 60 obese patients with apnea that, again, claimed to find a statistically significant effect between hypnosis and weight loss. However, the study shows that the results were small and clinically insignificant. In addition, they indicate that it is possible that he had not maintained adequate control of hypnotherapy, so the results are quite questionable.

As we can see, the research is too old, not very significant and doubtful, to be able to indicate that hypnosis has some kind of effect on weight loss. Neither as an individual treatment, nor in combination with other treatments. It would take a lot more research and much more updated.

Hypnosis Successes in Problems and Illnesses

Overweight, losing weight

Eating addiction (compulsive eating, the thoughts revolve around food)

addictive preferences, e.g. very strong appetite for chocolate, sweets, sweet drinks, carbohydrates

lack of or greatly delayed satiety

Eating-crushing addiction (Bulimia nervosa)

Compulsion to chew and spit out food

Eating attacks with addictive hunger attacks (binge eating disorder)

Eating at night (sometimes in a sleep-like state

Problems to accept one's own body

little motivation to move

Aversion to various foods

CHAPTER 2:

Is It Possible to Hypnotize Yourself?

We, as a whole, essentially need time to unwind, to dream, to imagine. It is refreshing to the physical body and restoring to the soul. At the point when we practice our hypnosis, it offers us simply that: an exceptionally close to home time to animate and enhance our mind and body. The training is done essentially. You don't require anything over an agreeable and safe spot.

Hypnosis Techniques

Getting ingested in your considerations and thoughts is that delicate excursion into the focal point of yourself called "going into a stupor." The straightforward methods of self-hypnosis incorporate going into a daze, deepening the daze, utilizing that daze state to give messages and recommendations to the mind-body, and coming out of the daze.

Subconscious Mind (Or Unconscious Mind)

This is the bit of our mind that performs capacities and procedures beneath our reasoning mindfulness. It is the mind of the body. It inhales us, digests, beats our hearts, and as a rule, deals with our automatic physical procedures for us. It can likewise instruct us to pick a bit of new mango rather than chocolate cake, to quit eating when we are full, or to appreciate a stroll in the recreation center.

Going into Trance

At the point when you are utilizing the stupor take a shot at the sound, I will be your guide as you go into a daze. I will utilize a daze enlistment strategy that you will discover quieting and centering. You have most likely observed the swinging watch technique in motion pictures, which is thirty-five years of training I have never observed anybody use, yet there is a wide range of approaches to concentrate on going into a stupor. You may gaze at a spot on the divider, utilize a breathing procedure, or utilize dynamic body unwinding. You will hear an assortment of acceptance strategies on the stupor work sound. They are just the prompts or the signs that you are providing for yourself to state, "I am going into a daze" or "I will do my hypnosis currently." Going into stupor can likewise be thought of as "letting yourself dream ...

intentionally." You are letting yourself become consumed in your contemplations and thoughts, exceptionally ingested, and permitting yourself to imagine or envision what you want as accomplished and genuine. There is no "going under." Instead, there is a beautiful encounter of going inside.

Deepening the Trance

Deepening your stupor causes you to become increasingly invested in your contemplations, thoughts, and experience. This is finished with dynamic unwinding: going "deeper and deeper inside ..." with pictures or scenes, or by checking a number arrangement, for instance. We like to propose that as you hear the checking from ten to zero, you make a vertical symbolism that is related to going deeper, for example, a way driving da mountain or into a rich green valley. As you hear me tallying, you can picture or envision going all the more deeply into a scene or spot that is considerably progressively pleasant and agreeable to you. This is the thing that we mean by "deepening the stupor."

Cognizant Mind

This is the "thinking mind" or the piece of the mind that gives us our mindfulness or feeling of knowing and oversees our deliberate capacities. For instance, our cognizant mind takes that second bit of pie at the meal, swipes the check card at the market, and moves the fork to our mouth.

The Betty Erickson Method

Betty Erickson developed this hypnosis technique. Although Betty wasn't a hypnotist, she understood of how our visual-auditory-kinesthetic systems influenced our world in a trance state. This technique has become increasingly popular in the world of hypnosis. This hypnosis technique can be used to relieve stress or any other self-hypnosis you would like to do.

The basic principles:

They are all thoughts in the form of images, full of sounds and emotions.

When we visualize, we think of all possible scenarios. We imagine how it is now, how we want it to be, and what it will be like in the future. This is simply a mixture of images that are already stored in the brain.

In the same way, our thoughts are associated with sounds, which are also the result of information stored in our minds, such as songs and sounds we imagine, speak, or hear. These sounds also include background noises and sounds we make when in dialogue with ourselves and others.

Emotions are the third way we think. These could be what we've experienced before or what we want to try or experience. Although our conscious mind uses these three, more often, only one is dominant. Therefore, for someone who associates his thoughts with sounds, he will not be as successful if he mainly uses visuals.

Before you move on to self-hypnosis, you may want to set goals for what you want to happen. Once you're ready, follow these steps.

Step 1: Get comfortable.

Sit or lie down in a quiet and comfortable position.

Relax your mind and body and feel yourself begin to wander in a state of relaxation. Let yourself in for a bit while staying on top of the outside world and keeping your eyes open, but you start to sleep.

Step 2: focus on something you are seeing.

Shadows moving across the wall or unique surroundings motifs can provide something unique to see. Be aware of what you see and become aware of it. Do it three different times, with three different objects.

Step 3: focus on something you are listening to

This could be the sound of your breathing, the wind brushing against the windows, or the hum of the air conditioner. Find three different things and observe them and bring them to your knowledge.

Step 4: focus on something you feel.

Maybe it's the movement of muscles along the joints, the gap between the shoulder blades, the weight of the feet on the floor, or the weight of the body on the chair. Consider three things and become aware of them.

Step 5: Continue with two things, then one thing.

Repeat steps 2-4, and this time, you will see two things, hear two things and feel two things. So, do the same for one thing.

Step 6: Close your eyes and go inward.

Allow yourself to go inward and relax and feel slightly drifting. This is a calm and peaceful state where you can simply let it go.

Step 7: imagine a new or old show

This could be what you saw before, or it could be something completely new. Imagine something you can see. Maybe it's a purple elephant, maybe it's a soothing blue light, or perhaps it's the sight of a ship taking off.

Step 8: imagine an old or new sound

You can create a sound, or it can be something you are already familiar with. An example is that you can hear the sound of an animal in nature, or a spacecraft suspended in space or the relaxing rain that falls on a group of leaves.

Step 9: imagine an old or new feeling

Become aware of something you've noticed before, or perhaps something you want to pay more attention to, such as how your breathing feels when it enters your lungs and the relaxation around your clavicle when you exhale.

Step 10: now, you are in hypnosis!

In this hypnotic state, you can make suggestions or just relax and let the ideas take effect that you had in mind before starting the session. Only trust that your mind is letting suggestions circulate: the more you can get carried away, the easier your ideas will take root inside.

Step 11: emerge

Say to yourself, "As I count from 1 to 5, I shall emerge with a great sense of energy, feeling refreshed and relaxed."

So, count from 1 to 5, allowing as much time as your body needs to make it real for you.

Benson Method

Benson can be widely credited for demystifying meditation and helping to bring it into the mainstream by changing the name of meditation to "Response to Relaxation." His studies have been able to show that meditation promotes better health. People who meditate regularly experience lower stress levels, greater well-being, and can even lower blood pressure levels and resting heart rate.

In his book, The Response to Relaxation, Dr. Benson describes the scientific benefits of relaxation, explaining that regular relaxation response practice can be an effective treatment for a wide range of stress-related ailments.

The relaxation response is the opposite reaction to the "fight" response. The relaxation response practice is beneficial as it neutralizes the physiological effects of stress and the fight-or-flight response.

It is normal for people experiencing the fight/flight response to describe uncomfortable physiological changes, such as muscle tension, headache, stomach pain, rapid heartbeat, and shallow breathing.

The relaxation response is an effective way to deactivate the fight/flight response and return the body to pre-stress levels.

There are multiple ways to elicit the relaxation response. Pure relaxation can be achieved by moving away from daily thinking and choosing a word, sound, phrase, sentence, or concentrating on your breathing and focusing on it.

Steps for an explicit relaxation response

Sit quietly in a comfortable position.

Close your eyes

Breathe through your nose. Become aware of your breathing. Breathe out, say the word "one" calmly to yourself.

Continue for 10-20 minutes. You can open your eyes to see the time, but you cannot use an alarm clock. When you are finished, sit quietly for a few minutes, initially with your eyes closed and then with your eyes open. Don't get up for a few minutes.

CHAPTER 3:

Reprogramming Starting from The Mind

Find a peaceable place to sit or lie down for complete relaxation then breathe and pay attention. Notice as the air tides in through your nostrils and how your belly buzzes to the maximum and gently falls back to your spine as you breathe out. Allow gravity to hold you securely in place. Breathe as naturally as you can. Do not force your breathing and take notice if your breath is quick or slow and steady.

Think of something that makes you feel happy and peaceful. Say to yourself, "I am thankful to be alive. I am secure and safe. I am confident and pure." Pay attention to your heart now. As you say these words to yourself, feel them deep within you. Give these statements positive energy and feed them with love. "I love myself; I can do anything I put my mind to. I trust that my brain, body, and soul are capable of providing me with what I desire most in life."

Breathe in now and fill your mind and soul with love and warmth. Imagine as you breathe in that there is a radiant light that fills your lungs before rapidly escaping your body. This light gives your patience, it gives you strength, and it provides you with the ambition and motivation to tackle the barriers that stand in your way. Breathe out naturally and notice as your body becomes heavier. With every breath that flows out, let go of negative thoughts; push those thoughts aside. You are good enough. You can do this. You are loved. You are special. Breathe out and release all of the tension that holds you back now. What other people believe and what you think are two different things. Say this now, "I believe in myself."

Count your breaths now. As you breathe in, breathe with your belly and count. One, two, three, four, and five. When you let go of this breath, make sure it is steady and slow. Breathe out, two, three, four, five. You are accepting this positive light to vibrate through your entire being. You are letting go of all the negativity that holds you back. Breathe in one, two, three, four. Breathe out one, two, three, four. And inhale for one, "I am happy," two, "I am strong," three, "I am kind," four, "I am brave," five, "I am driven to succeed." Breathe out now. You are counting your breath from one to five slow and steady. Positivity embraces you now; you feel light and in complete control. Nothing can disturb you; nothing can bring you down; you are perfect the way you are. Repeat this step until you are ready to watch your thoughts flow in and out.

Bring focus to your inner thoughts now. What pops into your mind? If you have any negative thoughts, let them be there as long as they want to be without judging them. Watch them, and then let them go. With every in-breath, notice your thoughts pop in without judgment. These thoughts are neither positive nor negative. When you breathe out, just let go of all hostility and anger you might be holding. Let it escape into the universe and breathe in, one, two, three, four, five; you are accepting all honesty and trust within yourself that you can make it through anything. "I am resilient. I am beautiful. I am a leader."

If you notice any negative thoughts, just see them and replace them with positive, self-loving thoughts.

Breaking Barriers

Make sure that you are in a place where you are completely comfortable and will not be disturbed for at least thirty minutes. Have the room you are inset to a comforting temperature and make sure that the lights are low. Adjust your body so that your shoulders are relaxed, your arms are lying on either side of you, and your palms are facing the ceiling. You want to become as comfortable and relaxed as you can so that your focus is not on your body but on the meditation. Gently close your eyes and take a deep breath inward until you can no longer breathe in. Exhale slowly and steadily so that all of the air escapes your lungs. Repeat these two more times.

Notice how your mind and body are relaxing into this guided exercise now. Breathe naturally now and bring your attention to your breath. Notice as the air fills your lungs and escapes as quickly as it entered. Breathing is something we do every day that we often take for granted. It's one of the many gifts that life gives us. Just be mindful of this moment you are in right now. Don't worry if your mind wanders; that's natural. There is no wrong way to do this. Put trust in yourself that right now, you are not performing; you don't have to be perfect.

Bring your attention to your body and your weight now. Visualize in your mind what you look like and try not to judge yourself too harshly. You are who you are, no matter what you look like or how you feel about that. Erase the tension and negativity from your mind; just be present with yourself right now.

Say to yourself,

"I am beautiful. I am strong. I can do this. I will lose weight, and I will not let anyone or anything stand in my way. The only opinion I will accept is what I think and feel about myself. At this moment and in my future moments, I believe that I am beautiful just the way that I am."

Let your breath suck in all these thoughts and have your mind believe everything you tell yourself as if it was your last wish on Earth.

As you visualize your weight right now, I would like you to imagine that you are at the starting line of a race. There are people just like you are competing for success.

Say to yourself

"I got this. I will not give up. I will succeed, and I will make it to the finish line. I will conquer my fears and overcome every obstacle that stands in my way."

In the background, you hear a coach shout, "Ready, get set..." Bring your awareness to your breath again. Inhale deeply and as you breathe in, get yourself fully committed and ready to take your first step toward losing weight. "Go!" Breathe out and visualize your feet, taking that first, second, and third step forward. Feel the pressure of your body press down on your legs and carry you forward. You realize this is hard, but you don't give up. You continue to jog ahead. Repeat this – "I know I can, I know I can, I know I can. I won't give up; I can do this."

You are now coming up to a bicycle, and as you get on it you feel the bike hold your weight. You will not fall. Put your feet on the pedals and start cycling. As you cycle, you continue faster and faster. Your heart is racing from the much-needed exercise. You feel good. Your lungs begin to hurt, but you push yourself as you notice the wind flying through your hair. Notice the droplets of sweat cool your skin. You got this. You are coming to a curve in the course now. Turn your bike and follow the path to the finish line. As you look back, you can see people just like yourself competing to finish, and there are a few behind you and a few ahead of you. While exercising, take a steady breath in and push it out forcefully. You should hear a pushing sound coming from your pursed lips. Inhale and say, "I got this, I won't give up. I will succeed." You are coming to the finish line now, but the course isn't over yet. As you cross the finish line, you get off your bike in third place. Way to go!

Bring your attention now to your breath. You are breathing heavily, your heart is racing, your chest hurts, but it's a euphoric feeling. You feel free; you broke out of the cycle and crossed the finish line. As you take a look down your body, you notice your body has become thinner. There is a scale in front of you on the sidelines; you've lost ten pounds. The feeling you are experiencing at this very moment is breathtaking, so you want to try it again. Trust that your body knows you and what to do. Trust in yourself that you will get through this.

You get ready again and wait to hear the coach. Take a deep breath in for a count of five. When I count down, you can start your course. Five, four, three, two, one, and go! Let out your breath and feel your legs carry your ten-pounds-lighter body. This time it's a little more comfortable than the first round. Your breath quickens, and your heart speeds up. You can do this.

Say to yourself,

"I will complete this course. I am strong enough to conquer any barrier that stands in my way. This is hard, but nothing easy is worth doing. I got this."

In front of you now is a blow-up house with a wide opening. You crawl through this opening and are covered by colorful plastic balls. They are flying at you from all angles, and it becomes hard to see. Soon, you are swimming through these balls moving forward. You push these balls aside, and as you look up; you see another opening. "I got this,"

You say to yourself.

"I will make it through, and nothing can stop me now." As you reach the opening, you crawl through and are entirely on your stomach. You are in a narrow hole that you must army-crawl through to reach the end. Take in a deep breath now. Nothing scares you. Nothing can get to you. Imagine this hole the way everyone else bullied you or picked on you. You might have felt small, or enclosed, singled out, or trapped.

CHAPTER 4:

Is It Possible to Use Hypnosis to Eliminate Food Addictions?

Food fixation has numerous clinical names, and people may have numerous instances of this occurring, for example, overeating happens when people plan to devour an over the top amount of nourishment often. In a brief span, frequently thoughtlessly, a gorge eater will, in general, devour a large number of calories, and these gorges have serious wellbeing outcomes. Regularly the desire to gorge is unreasonable entrancing encourages us to deal with and manage these inclinations.

On the opposite side, habitual gorging is practically identical. Enthusiastic overeaters are much of the time overpowered by yearnings, most often for sugar, milk, or carbs. Furthermore, as per the National Center for Eating Disorders, they feel an absence of order over their yearnings. Entrancing instructs us to recognize yearnings, reinventing the subliminal to be progressively steady in vanquishing indulge desires.

A few people are at last calling themselves sugar addicts or carb addicts. Their desires are for specific sustenance, and these unfortunate choices, they can't kick their longings. For instance, the entrance of sugar fixation can help us reframe how the subliminal perspectives sugar, and essentially can enable us to diminish our longings.

Despite the kind of compulsion, numerous sustenance addicts have comparative side effects:

- Fast eating

- Continue to consume food despite not feeling hungry

- Secretly eating

- Feeling blame or regret for indulging and

- Feeling constrained or "spurred" to eat

So, What Triggers This Unfortunate Relationship With Food?

The underlying drivers of our sustenance addictions are overwhelmingly in the intuitive personality. For example, we have been adapted to append positive associations with certain sustenance sorts, or overeating or gorging, and these affiliations are profoundly established in the subliminal.

How Our Thoughts Contribute

The issue isn't over-utilization, gorging, or serious longings. The issue is the unfavorable reasoning examples that drive us to make undesirable eating choices. These affiliations are shockingly, profoundly imbued. We spent our lives molding ourselves for unfortunate eating.

Gatherings, weddings, hot treats from grandmother, we found that our companions are sugar tidbits and greasy sustenance. Huge numbers of us use them to remunerate ourselves, mend fatigue or nervousness, and when we feel focused on, a few of us eat.

What's more, all the time, automatically, our yearnings are caused. We're encountering anxiousness and stress! We get into the bureau and eat without truly contemplating why. Frequently we don't significantly consider our intuitive personalities the area where the study shows that 85-95% of cerebrum movement lives. What's more, this is the cerebrum district where there is sustenance fixation.

Our intuitive thoughts are programmed, and a lifetime of experience has fortified them. For example, we may have found solace in sustenance after a horrendous youth case, discovering that nourishment desensitized feelings of agony or disgrace. We change to nourishment for comfort, as should be obvious!

Positive events can likewise be connected to our tensions. Envision this: Someone could connect sweetly with grandma preparing. Thusly, in their inner minds, desserts are associated with adoration and wellbeing. That is the reason in enthusiastic conditions, or when we're pushed, such a large number of us go to nourishment, we need comfort!

The amazing news: you can retrain the intuitive. Spellbinding normally and proficiently empowers us to keep up the subliminal. Furthermore, numerous conditions that are made by unfortunate examples of intuition, for example, uneasiness and stress, have been appeared to help.

We can likewise utilize entrancing to get to the subliminal and give new, increasingly valuable information to this astounding information storehouse. Consider it destroying weeds to plant crisp sound seeds. We may reframe how we accept low-quality nourishment, for example, and elevate the subliminal to search for and ache for more beneficial choices.

Can Hypnotherapy be used for Food Addiction?

At this point, you have a thought of how spellbinding helps: it engages us to know about our yearnings and empowers the psyche to consider sustenance. Yet, how does that work correctly?

Here is an outline of a portion of the better nourishment dependence entrancing focuses and a portion of the numerous ways it can engage us to lead a more advantageous life.

Careful eating

There is a tantamount manifestation in practically all sustenance addictions: we frequently over-eat without speculation. It's turning into an impulse, and something we're not purposely considering. We can show the brain to be progressively aware of our desires, how complete we feel, and the genuine demonstration of eating with mesmerizing for cautious eating. Mesmerizing of cautious eating empowers us to recognize hunger yearnings and physical feelings and to think about eating. We are picking up power over nourishment and our yearning.

Breaking Habitual Thoughts

Common reasoning winds up reactionary and negative very frequently. Furthermore, regularly, these thoughts trigger our longings or over-utilization. You may confront a distressing condition at work, and as opposed to breathing and saying it's everything going to be OK, you start believing you're under-qualified, or the pressure transforms into tension. We can't discharge our sustenance addictions without disposing of these spiraling reasoning examples. Entrancing empowers us to recover control of our thoughts and make our inner mind a solid partner.

Gastric Band Hypnosis

Hypnosis deals with the natural state of awareness. This is typically embarked in a clinical environment to assist people in making positive improvements and changes in their lives.

Hypnotherapy for Weight Loss

Lots of people suggest that if you desire fat-burning through natural means, you must think about trying weight management hypnotherapy. So just how does this fat burn hypnosis hypnotherapy function in the weight management field? Research studies exposed that weight control using hypnosis works, but the stomach band hypnotherapy is also confirmed to be extra reliable.

Stomach band hypnosis is not valid for everyone, and this weight control hypnosis functions best on people with a proper state of mind. Its own merits in determining each weight-reduction situation for suitable viability.

The following are five things you probably do not recognize regarding Gastric band hypnosis. Keep reading to aim and also find out what you require to discover this weight-loss alternative.

1. You Do not Have Gastric Band Fitted

This appears to be among the distinct points to cover. Some people are puzzled regarding the stomach band hypnosis technique and also the real clinical procedures offered privately. Hypnoband is the usual stomach band hypnosis method, and this does not involve surgical treatments.

The hypnotherapy is a non-invasive kind of weight management using suggestions and cognitive-behavioral therapies to attain desired results.

2. Will This Work for You?

The gastric band hypnosis is, in some way, reliant on you. For the best outcomes, you should completely commit to losing weight in your heart and wellness. This weight reduction service is not really for people looking for someone controlling them. You are the only key to your fat-burning success.

Many individuals can slim down if they are prepared to change their total lifestyle and behaviors. It likewise assists to have a support system right in your very own home. If you're always triggered to consume improper meals, gastric band hypnotherapy can have straight effects on your weight loss results, particularly. This one will work for you if you are serious regarding shedding weight.

3. Is stomach band hypnosis assured to Make You Lose More Weight than other methods?

Since various aspects may influence the results, no clinical side effect may alter results. Bear in mind that with any kind of hypnosis, the concern of stopping smoking cigarettes and even more are results reliant on individuals. If the person is not 100% devoted, no form of hypnosis will work.

You need to recognize that the mind is an active and complicated body organ through undertaking this gastric band hypnosis, you will undoubtedly be equipping yourself with required devices to transform your old and undesirable eating behaviors completely. Treatment is generally intended to assist individuals in turning habits and dropping weight.

4. what to expect?

This usually consists of evaluation sessions and long-hour sessions of therapy. An ethical hypnotherapist will take a complete breakdown of your clinical and dietary history before waging treatment. Throughout the very first therapy, you'll be introduced to hypnosis the state of even more enhanced discovering wherein; you will feel ultimately tranquil and also un-winded.

In the following session, you will certainly then be presented to gastric band hypnosis, and also your hypnotherapist will use a fit digital gastric band for excellent results.

5. What is the Cost?

There is genuinely no set price, and also generally, the extra successful the therapists are, the higher the price, and the more they will bill since they can back up their insurance claims and, after that, verify results.

A gastric band is a versatile silicone gadget utilized in the weight reduction clinical procedure. The group is established around the top location of the stomach to make little pouch over the gizmo. This limits the process of food that can be kept in the belly, making it hard to consume considerable amounts.

The gastric band's objective is to confine the measure of foods one can consume, making them feel full upon eating a bit to equip weight decrease. Like any treatment, fitting a stomach band still comes with risks, so people intend to reduce weight still require to be mindful of this.

A gastric band can be made use of to help individuals properly drop weight without any risks that come with surgical treatments. There is a two-pronged approach that usually made use by hypnotherapists. They will take a better look at identifying the root triggers of a person's emotional eating.

Using Hypnotherapy, the specialist can urge you to bear in mind long-overlooked encounters, including foods that could be intuitively affecting you now.

By making use of the relaxation methods, the hypnotherapists will position you in a state of hypnosis. Under this relaxed stage, your subconscious becomes extra open to tips and also at this price; hypnotherapists will make recommendations right into your sub-conscious. With the Gastric Band Hypnotherapy, this specific idea is that you've had the band fitted, and given that the mind is so powerful, so as soon as your account approves this pointer, your practices will change appropriately. Along with suitable this stomach band, suggestions that border behavior and also self-confidence will trigger you to dedicate with a pleasing way of life adjustments.

Additionally, informing yourself concerning exercise and nourishment is suggested to promote physical health and wellness.

This therapy includes fat burning hypnosis that will certainly aid you to drop those added pounds. This can likewise belong to your weight loss strategy that includes working out, diet programs, and also coaching. When you enter into hypnosis hypnotic trance, you need to be extra responsive to recommendations that might consist of practices changes that better assist you in reducing weight.

CHAPTER 5:

Keep Motivation High

Motivation is one of the most powerful tools in creating permanent change. Your motivation is based on what you believe. And as you are probably aware, belief is scarcely based on your concrete reality. In essence, you believe things because of how you see them, feel them, hear them, smell them, and so forth. You can program your mind by taking feelings from one of your experiences and connecting those feelings to a different experience. Let us look at how you can remain motivated to lose weight:

Establish Where You Are Now

You should take a full-length picture of yourself at the present as a push mechanism from your current position, as well as for comparison later on. Two primary factors are relevant to health. One is whether you like the image you see in the mirror and the second is how you feel. Do you have the energy to do what you wish, and are you feeling strong enough?

- Explore your reasons for wanting to lose weight. These are what will keep you going even when you don't feel like it.

- Assess your eating habits and establish your reasons for overeating or indulging in the wrong foods.

- It is assumed that you have the desire to get healthier and lose weight. Here, you state clearly and positively to yourself what you want, and then decide that you will accomplish it with persistence. Use the self-hypnosis routine explained above to drive this point into your subconscious mind.

- Determine your motivation for the desired results, and how you will know when you've accomplished the goal. How will you feel, what will you see, and what are you likely to hear when you achieve your goal?

- Devote the first session of self-hypnosis to making the ultimate decision about your weight. Note that you must never have any doubt in your mind about your challenge to lose weight.

- Plan your meals every day. Weigh yourself frequently to monitor your progress as well. However, do not be paranoid about weighing yourself as this can actually negatively affect your progress.

- Repeat to yourself every day that you are getting to your ideal weight, that you've developed new, sensible eating habits, and that you are no longer prone to temptation.

- Think positively and provide positive affirmations in your self-induced hypnotic state.

Tweak Your Lifestyle

Every little thing counts. This is an important thing to note if you want to lose weight and slim down. Making a few changes in your regular daily activities can help you burn more calories.

Walk more

Use the stairs instead of the escalator or elevator if you're just going up or down a floor or two.

Park your car a mile away from your destination and walk the rest of the way. You can also walk briskly to burn more calories.

During your rest day, make it more active by taking your dog for a long walk in the park.

If you need to travel a few blocks, save gas and avoid traffic by walking. For greater distances, dust off that old bike and pedal your way to your destination.

Watch how and what you eat

A big breakfast kicks your body into hypermetabolism mode so you should not skip the first meal of the day.

Brushing after a meal signals your brain that you've finished eating, making you crave less until your next scheduled meal.

If you need to get food from a restaurant, make your order to-go so you won't get tempted by their other offerings.

Plan your meals for the week, so you can count how many calories you are consuming in a day.

Make quick, healthy meals so you save time. There are thousands of recipes out there. Do some research.

Eat at a table, not in your car. Drive-thru food is almost always greasy and full of unhealthy carbohydrates.

Put more leaves, like arugula and alfalfa sprouts on your meals to give you more fiber and make you eat less.

Order the smallest meal size if you really need to eat fast food.

Start your meal with a vegetable salad. Dip the salad into the dressing instead of pouring it on.

For a midnight snack, munch on protein bars or just drink a glass of skim milk.

Eat before you go to the grocery to keep yourself from being tempted by food items that you don't really plan to buy.

Clean out your pantry by taking out food items that won't help you with your fitness goals.

The whole idea in the tweaks mentioned is that you should eat less and move more. You may be able to think of additional tweaks.

CHAPTER 6:

Weight Loss Tips

Befofe you can begin using meditations to do things such as help you burn fat, you need to make sure that you set yourself up properly for your meditation sessions. Each meditation is going to consist of you entering a deep state of relaxation, following a guided hypnosis, and then awakening yourself out of this state of relaxation. If done properly, you will find yourself experiencing the stages of changed mindset and changed behavior that follows the session.

In order to properly set yourself up for a meditation experience, you need to make sure that you have a quiet space where you can engage in your meditation. You want to be as uninterrupted as possible so that you do not stir awake from your meditation session. Aside from having a quiet space, you should also make sure that you are comfortable in the space that you will be in. For some of the meditations, I will share, you can be lying down or doing this meditation before bed so that the information sinks in as you sleep. For others, you are going to want to be sitting upright, ideally with your legs crossed on the floor, or with your feet planted on the floor as you sit in a chair. Staying in a sitting position, especially during morning meditations, will help you stay awake and increase your motivation. Laying down during these meditations earlier in the day may result in you draining your energy and feeling completely exhausted, rather than motivated. As a result, you may actually work against what you are trying to achieve.

Each of these meditations is going to involve a visualization practice; however, if you find that visualization is generally difficult for you, you can simply listen. The key here is to make sure that you keep as open of a mind as possible so that you can stay receptive to the information coming through these guided meditations.

Aside from all of the above, listening to low music, using a pillow or a small blanket, and dressing in comfortable loose clothing will all help you have better meditations. You want to make sure that you make these experiences the best possible so that you look forward to them and regularly engage in them. As well, the more relaxed and comfortable you are, the more receptive you will be to the information being provided to you within each meditation.

A Simple Daily Weight Loss Meditation

This meditation is an excellent simple meditation for you to use on a daily basis. It is a short meditation that will not take more than about 15 minutes to complete, and it will provide you with excellent motivation to stick to your weight loss regimen every single day. You should schedule time in your morning routine to engage in this simple daily weight loss meditation every single day. You can also complete it periodically throughout the day if you find your motivation dwindling or your mindset regressing. Over time, you should find that using it just once per day is plenty.

Because you are using this meditation in the morning, make sure that you are sitting upright with a straight spine so that you are able to stay engaged and awake throughout the entire meditation. Laying down or getting too comfortable may result in you feeling more tired, rather than more awake, from your meditation. Ideally, this meditation should lead to boosted energy as well as improved fat burning abilities within your body.

The Meditation

Start by gently closing your eyes and drawing your attention to your breath. As you do, I want you to track the next five breaths, gently and intentionally lengthening them to help you relax as deeply as you can. With each breath, breathe in to the count of five and out to the count of seven.

Now that you are starting to feel more relaxed, I want you to draw your awareness into your body. First, become aware of your feet. Feel your feet relaxing deeply, as you visualize any stress or worry melting away from your feet. Now, become aware of your legs. Feel any stress or worry melting away from your legs as they begin to relax completely. Next, become aware of your glutes and pelvis, allowing any stress or worry to simply fade away as they completely relax. Now, become aware of your entire torso, allowing any stress or worry to melt away from your torso as it relaxes completely. Next, become aware of your shoulders, arms, hands, and fingers. Allow the stress and worry to melt away from your shoulders, arms, hands, and fingers as they relax completely. Now, let the stress and worry melt away from your neck, head, and face. Feel your neck, head, and face relaxing as any stress or worry melts away completely.

As you deepen into this state of relaxation, I want you to take a moment to visualize the space in front of you. Imagine that in front of you, you are standing there looking back at yourself. See every inch of your body as it is right now standing before you, casually, as you simply observe yourself. While you do, see what parts of your body you want to reduce fat in so that you can create a healthier, stronger body for yourself. Visualize the fat in these areas of your body, slowly fading away as you begin to carve out a healthier, leaner, and stronger body underneath. Notice how effortlessly this extra fat melts away as you continue to visualize yourself becoming a healthier and more vivacious version of yourself.

Now, I want you to visualize what this healthier, leaner version of yourself would be doing. Visualize yourself going through your typical daily routine, except from the perspective of your healthier self. What would you be eating? When and how would you be exercising? What would you spend your time doing? How do you feel about yourself? How different do you feel when you interact with the people around you, such as your family and your co-workers? What does life feel like when you are a healthier, leaner version of you?

Spend several minutes visualizing how different your life is now that your fat has melted away. Feel how natural it is for you to enjoy these healthier foods, and how easy it is for you to moderate your cravings and indulgences when you choose to treat yourself. Notice how easy it is for you to engage in exercise and how exercise feels enjoyable and like a wonderful hobby, rather than a chore that you have to force yourself to commit to every single day. Feel yourself genuinely enjoying life far more, all because the unhealthy fats that were weighing you down and disrupting your health have faded away. Notice how easy it was for you to get here, and how easy it is for you to continue to maintain your health and wellness as you continue to choose better and better choices for you and your body.

Feel how much you respect your body when you make these healthier choices, and how much you genuinely care about yourself. Notice how each meal and each exercise feels like an act of self-care, rather than a chore you are forcing yourself to engage in. Feel how good it feels to do something for you. For your wellbeing.

When you are ready, take that visualization of yourself and send the image out really far, watching it become nothing more than a spec in your field of awareness. Then, send it out into the ether, trusting that your subconscious mind will hold onto this vision of yourself and work daily on bringing this version of you into your current reality.

Now, awaken back into your body where you sit right now. Feel yourself feeling more motivated, more energized, and more excited about engaging in the activities that are going to improve your health and help you burn your fat. As you prepare to go about your day, hold onto that visualization and those feelings that you had of yourself, and trust that you can have this wonderful experience in your life. You can do it!

CHAPTER 7:

How Hypnosis Accelerates Weight Loss

How Hypnosis helps you Achieve Rapid Weight Loss

During hypnosis, your mind becomes open to any suggestions. In fact, studies have shown that when in the hypnotic state, your brain is likely to experience interesting changes, which allows learning about the information you are receiving without having to think critically or consciously.

In this state, you are always detached from your conscious mind, thus, you don't interrupt your thoughts with the question about what you are hearing. And this is how hypnosis helps with the breaking down of barriers that prevent you from shedding off weight.

In hypnotherapy, repetition is the key to success. This explains why many hypnotherapists provide you with self-hypnosis recordings, which you own to listen to repeatedly. The barriers in the brain are always very strong, and only through repeated hypnosis can you untangle yourself from the convictions.

Hypnosis teaches the mind how to think differently about eating and food. The suggestions above can help you achieve the following:

Control Food Cravings

Weight loss hypnotic technique can help you to detach yourself from cravings and isolate yourself from unhealthy foods. For instance, during hypnosis, you might be asked to visualize how you will send away the cravings. Suggestions can help in reframing cravings and teach you how to manage them in an effective manner.

Success

Expectations of an individual dictate his/her reality. With the expectation of success, we are apt to take the steps necessary to attain success. Hypnosis can plant this seed of success in your mind, thus, giving you the unconscious power to keep yourself on course.

Positivity

Nobody likes negativity, and our brains are no different. Negative thoughts can spoil your ability and dedication to lose weight. Through hypnosis, you will become aware of the foods that you "can't eat." These foods do not help your body or health in any way. Thus, hypnotherapy will make you understand that you are not punishing yourself by abstaining from these foods, but you are doing that to improve your overall being.

Preparing for Relapse

Our minds have been trained to think that relapsing from a journey or goal is a sinful act, as it is a reason to give up. However, hypnosis gives us the chance of relapsing differently. The relapse becomes an opportunity to examine what went wrong, and learn from it, then get prepared for any future temptation.

Modifying Behaviors

We can only achieve big goals by taking small steps at a time. Hypnosis empowers us to take the step for these small changes, which eventually result in bigger goals. For instance, when you always reward yourself with high-calorie content and sugary foods, you will, over time, choose a healthier reward through hypnosis.

What to Expect in a Hypnotherapy session?

Hypnotherapy sessions can vary in methodology and length depending on the practitioner. However, on average, a session takes lasts for 45 minutes to 60 minutes but may go for as long as 3 to 4 hours for weight loss patients. The general procedure entails lying down, relaxing with eyes closed, and letting the therapist guide you through suggestions, which can help you reach your goals.

Through the history of your weight loss journey, a hypnotherapist is able to train your mind towards what is healthy food and away from unhealthy foods. Although you will be in an unconscious state of mind, the process does not make you do what you are not willing to. Someone in a hypnotic trance will literally be between being asleep and wide awake. Thus, you are fully aware of the suggestions made by the hypnotherapist, and as such can control or even stop the process.

CHAPTER 8:

The Power of Affirmations

This simple and clear, effective method to produce weight loss affirmations is just what you're looking for when you're ready to reach your ideal weight, get more energy every day, and get higher self-esteem.

Set a goal.

First and foremost, in generating positive affirmations about weight loss is identifying a specific target weight at which you feel confident about achieving it. Many people opt for weight loss simply because they want to lose weight. The problem with this method of thought is that our minds were programmed to believe they should lose something as being evil. And when the subconscious mind mentions weight loss, it automatically connects weight loss to a negative feeling, in addition to a depressed state of mind arising from issues with depression.

No-one wants to lose weight... And they want to hit their target weight, so that is a primary so essential difference if you're going to achieve a rapid weight loss.

TIP: A smart idea would be to contact your doctor or use an accurate target weight calculator to support the decision process for the optimal weight. When predicting, or because you think this is the only weight you could be comfortable with, you can by no way settle on a target weight.

Decide How to Change Yourself.

Affirmations of healthy weight loss or diet pills alone won't help you achieve fast weight loss. You have to make improvements in your diet and levels of behavior which have already been compounded by the issues of depression. Efforts to find a way around this and to achieve rapid weight loss would take a toll on the body that doesn't make it worth. Decide precisely what adjustments are needed to accomplish your aim, in addition to choosing the ideal weight. In doing so, you would be giving your rational mind a specific set of behaviors to cause the body to take. It can also help with the struggles you're experiencing with depression because it allows the mind something different to understand.

Construct Your Assertions.

Finally, after finding out your ideal weight and understanding what adjustments you can make to accomplish this, build up your affirmations. You would need to follow four fundamental rules to do this:

Action focused implies that from step two, the affirmations discuss a specific work. In other words: "I consume more nutritious foods and therefore achieve my ideal weight by reconditioning my metabolism"; "I achieve my ideal weight by engaging in strength exercise and cardiovascular exercise"; "Because of my dedication to good nutrition and an active lifestyle, I experience improved energy and self-esteem". Then you should write them down. Lastly, you put these assumptions to work...

Rehearsal daily.

Reconditioning your subconscious mind and maintenance, your body follows a standard set of beliefs and, if practiced, that will assist with your struggles with depression. For starters, if you wanted to go to the gym a few times, you wouldn't expect to achieve lasting effects on yourself. You must, therefore, devote yourself to regular practice, and adapt it as a part of your lifestyle ... And most significantly, embrace it and you might even overcome your problems with depression. Say them aloud once every morning and evening as soon as you have your weight reduction affirmations made.

This is the secret of preparing your unconscious mind for quick weight loss by affirmations of successful weight loss and is a solution to your issues with depression.

Strong assertions are a handy tool for helping you lose weight. At best, it can be difficult when you're trying to lose weight, particularly when you're experiencing depression, but you don't feel that comfortable about yourself. Being overweight can trigger all kinds of negative emotions which make it more challenging to stay motivated. Everything you say to yourself affects the conditions and circumstances considerably. Yes, most people don't know how destructive their habits of thought are. Have you ever glimpsed your body in the mirror and felt your heart sink? What if you say "I'm so fat and abominable"? These two are very typical examples of negative self-talking. Negative self-talk is both a deadly zapper of inspiration and an awful thing for your overall self-esteem. Losing weight requires perseverance and determination, and you owe it to yourself to do whatever it takes to remain optimistic and motivated if you want to succeed in the long term. And what exactly are statements? They are often confident statements written or spoken in the present tense, reflecting on the result or goal you want to accomplish.

The first step in using positive affirmations is to focus on what you want to accomplish, and then make a series of comments that represent that aim as if it was happening right now. And if you aim to lose weight, for example, you might say:

- "I can easily reach and sustain my ideal weight";

- "I love and value my body".

Here are some more instances of positive weight-loss claims:

- "Weight loss comes easily to me".

- "I can meet my weight loss goals".

- "I get weight loss every day".

- "I love the savor of healthy food".

- "I supervise how much I eat".

- "I enjoy exercising, and it makes me feel excellent".

- "I am getting fitter and healthier by exercising".

- "I'm continually cultivating more balanced eating habits".

- "I get slimmer with every day".

- "I am looking fantastic and feeling fine".

- "I can quickly achieve and sustain my ideal weight".

- "I love and care for my body".

- "I deserve to have a lean, happy, beautiful mass".

- "I love to exercise daily".

- "All I eat contributes to my health and well-being.

- "I only eat when I'm hungry".

- "I can see myself clearly at my ideal weight".

Once you've created your positive affirmations, you have to set aside each one for some time.

There are quite a few ways you can do that. You may pick one sentence and say it out loud ten times in the morning and ten times in the evening, or you may want to reiterate it to yourself when you think about it all day long. Picture that happening right now when you reaffirm your sentence: Imagine yourself doing or thinking about the nature of what your sentence says. Keep it as accurate in your mind's eye as possible. Your subconscious produces a mental blueprint as you visualize and imagine your target.

Try to make use of optimistic words that you feel confident with and that work for you. You have to tell them regularly (at least 3-4 times a day) with a real conviction for them to work. Please tell them when you wake up in the morning and the last thing before bedtime. If you can get time alone, it can be motivational to say them out loud. Write down your optimistic comments on some card and take them around with you at any time of the day for an immediate boost. You might even post them at your fridge, a brilliant way to help you think before snacking becomes unhealthy.

To build a habit, you have to say your positive affirmations regularly (each day) for at least 30 days. It's also essential that you get used to ejecting harmful thoughts as soon as they get into your brain. Make everyday use of positive affirmations for weight loss results, and look forward to a fresh look and a happy you.

How to Replace Your Negative Habits And Eating Patterns With Positive Ones?

There are several nuanced explanations on why people in their everyday lives establish unhealthy eating habits. Once it comes to actively and positively altering these behaviors, weight loss hypnosis operates by interrupting harmful practices and replacing them with new motivational ones. From how the mind affects the body, how fat and toxins are removed by consuming nutritious food and drinking clean water, how deep breathing stimulates the metabolism of the organs and how constant personal growth helps to achieve success.

To make a drastic shift in a body of people, changes must first be made within their minds. The subconscious mind still works to keep you stable and in line with your daily actions. That's why dieting alone sometimes isn't enough to lose the last extra pounds. Because thoughts in minds have a powerful impact on the body, and yet healthy weight loss and improved metabolism require new behavioral habits. That this occurs because it shakes the old thoughts and habits.

The number one explanation for overeating is to prevent mental distress or mask it. We need to learn to forgive ourselves and practice self-love for this purpose. Weight loss hypnosis allows us to accept a new self and release the old overweight habits by interrupting them and training them in new safe and beneficial patterns. If the old pattern is consuming sugar and fried foods, then a routine of eating fresh vegetables, nuts, seeds, berries and clean water needs to be the new trend. That is the first step on the journey.

They claim you are what you eat, and you finally are what you think about most of you. You begin by praising yourself with weight loss hypnosis, and then reinforce your new ideal slim self with optimistic thinking, positive emotions, and new eating habits such as consuming steamed vegetables, salads, and soups with every meal, instead of candies and snacks on nuts, seeds and berries. Eating naturally based foods and drinking plenty of fresh drinks will allow your body to quickly remove the fat and toxins that are stored in the tissues of your body. The aim is to remove the old addictions to food and sugar and give the body what it wants.

There is one new thing the body needs and desires, along with balanced foods and safe drinking water. Deep rhythmic breathing is a long-lived secret to success with hypnosis in weight loss and secure life. You fill the blood with oxygen by breathing deeply in and breathing out absolutely. When you exhale toxins, you activate the lymphatic system, the way the body removes waste. By developing a ritual of deep breathing for yourself, 5-10 minutes, three times a day, you can dramatically increase your metabolism and your strength. That one habit will alone change your life. Hypnotists consider these principalities and the following method the magic recipe in weight loss hypnosis.

Do you have some problem that you want to eliminate? Is your servant's habit, or is it your master? Are you aware that your actions eventually decide your future?

You don't just fall into the life you want, and you have to build what you want by taking steps in the direction of your goals, no matter what you may want in life.

Ask yourself some questions about the habits you have formed, and some are going to be good habits in that they are aligned with your beliefs, while other habits are unhelpful and do not serve your goals in life.

CHAPTER 9:

Love Yourself Always

The majority of individuals don't think very much about self-improvement. We'd love to assist you to indulge in such a notion and find out just how much you can enjoy yourself. It's a requirement for accepting and creating your ideal weight and everything else that's fantastic for you. Just being conscious of the idea of self-help can move you farther along on the way of enjoying yourself and accepting yourself as you are. Your character and character are aware of the way you're feeling on your own. If you harbor bitterness or remorse, or sense undeserving, these emotions operate contrary to enjoying yourself.

- How can you see your flaws?

- Can you blame yourself? Self-love and finding an error or depriving yourself repaint each other. It is tough to enjoy yourself if you frequently find error ultimately.

- Can you put attention on negative aspects of yourself?

- Can you end up making self-deprecating statements, such as "I am not intelligent enough to..." or even "I am not great enough to..."?

- Can you punish yourself or refuse yourself?

- Can you establish boundaries with individuals who represent your very own moral and ethical criteria and your values and beliefs?

- Look at the mirror. How do you feel about yourself? Can you smile or frown?

- Which are you about the continuum of self?

- Are you currently respectful and admiring?

- Are you critical and judgmental, or would you love yourself for that you are?

- Have you been caring and caring this individual who you see?

If you're ambivalent, then contemplate these concerns further. Be truthful with yourself. Have a conversation on your own. Take a sincere look at yourself. Do not just examine your own body; examine your wisdom, your soul, your own emotions, along with your own heart. Know that: By enjoying yourself, you love yourself. If there's something that you can't accept on your own, be aware you could change that idea, and alter it to make anything you want, such as your ideal weight.

How Does It Feel to Love Yourself?

Have a look at These features. Are these familiar to you? It is the way it should feel if you like yourself:

- You genuinely feel happy and accepting your world, even though you might not agree with everything within it.

- You're compassionate with your flaws or less-than-perfect behaviors, understanding that you're capable of improving and changing.

- You mercifully love compliments and feel joyful inside.

- You frankly see your flaws and softly accept them learn to alter them.

- You accept all of the goodness that comes your way.

- You honor the great qualities and the fantastic qualities of everybody around you.

- You look at the mirror and smile (at least all the period).

Many confuse self-love with becoming arrogant and greedy. But some individuals are so caught up in themselves they make the tag of being egotistical and thinking just of these. We do not find that as a healthful self-indulgent, however, as a character which isn't well balanced in enjoying itself love and loving others.

It isn't selfish to get things your way; however, it's egotistical to insist that everybody else can see them your way too. The Dalai Lama states, "If you do not enjoy yourself, then you can't love other people. You won't have the capacity to appreciate others. If you don't have any empathy on your own, then you aren't capable of developing empathy for others" Dr. Karl Menninger, a psychologist, states it this way: "Self-love isn't opposed to this love of different men and women. You can't truly enjoy yourself and get yourself a favor with no people a favor, and vice versa." We're referring to the healthiest type of self-indulgent, that simplifies the solution to accepting your best good.

Just take a better look at the way you see your flaws and blame yourself. Self-love and finding an error or depriving yourself aren't in any way compatible. If you deny enjoying yourself, you're in danger of paying too much focus on your flaws, that is a sort of self-loathing. You don't wish to place focus on negative aspects of yourself, for by keeping these ideas in your mind, you're giving them the psychological energy which brings that result or leaves it actual.

Self-love is positive energy. Blame, criticism, and faultfinding are energy. Self-hypnosis can help you utilize your mind-body to make new and much more loving ideas and beliefs on your own. It helps your mind-body create and take fluctuations in the patterns of feeling and thinking which have been for you for quite a while, and which aren't helpful for you. The trancework about the sound incorporates many positive suggestions to shift your ideas, emotions, and beliefs in alignment together with your ideal weight.

A Vital goal for all these positive hypnotic suggestions is the innermost feeling of enjoying yourself. If your self-loving feelings are constant with your ideal weight, then it is going to occur with increased ease. But if you harbor bitterness or remorse, or sense undeserving, these emotions operate contrary to enjoying yourself enough to think and take your ideal weight. Lucille Ball stated it well: "Love yourself first and everything falls in line" The hypnotic suggestions about the sound are directions for change led to the maximum "internal" degree of mind-body or unconscious. However, the "outer" changes in life action should also happen.

Many weight reduction methods you have been using might appear to be a lot of work. We suggest that by adopting a mindset that's without the psychological pressure related to "needing to," "bad or good," or even "simple or difficult," with no judgment in any way, the fluctuations could be joyous.

Yes, even joyous. It produces the whole journey of earning adjustments and shifting easier. The term "a labor of love" implies you enjoy doing this so much it isn't labor or responsibility. The "labor" of organizing a family feast in a vacation season, volunteering at a hospital or school, or even buying a gift for someone very particular can appear effortless. Here is the mindset that will assist you in following some weight loss methods. We invite you to place yourself in the situation of being adored.

You're doing so to you. Loving yourself eliminates the job, and that means it is possible to relish your advancement toward a lifestyle that encourages your ideal weight. Think about some action that you like to perform. Imagine yourself performing this action today. Notice that whenever you're doing something which you love to perform, you're feeling energized and beautiful, and some other attempt is evidenced by enjoyment. What is going on at these times is you see it absolutely "loving what you're doing." Sometimes, we recommend that you also find that as "enjoying yourself doing this." Maybe by directing more favorable attitude toward enjoying yourself, you'll end up enjoying what you're doing.

Lisa's Brimming Smile

After Lisa and Rick wed, both have been slender and appreciated active lifestyles which included softball and Pilates classes at the local gym. When their very first infant was first born, Lisa had obtained an additional fifteen lbs. From now, their infant came three decades later, and she had been twenty pounds' overweight. Depending on the demands of motherhood, she depended on fast-frozen foods, canned foods, and food to the table. Persistent sleep deprivation also maintained her power level reduced, and she can hardly keep up with the toddlers. Rick, a promising young company executive, took more and more duties on the job increasing the "ladder of success," indulging in company lunches, and even working late afternoon. He'd return home late; fall facing the TV and eat leftover pizza.

The youthful couple accepted their ancestral lifestyle but observed with dismay as their bodies grew tired and old beyond their years. However, they lasted. If their oldest boy entered astronomy, they became more upset. Small Ricky appeared to be the goal of each germfree, and he started to miss several days of college. If this was not enough, he also attracted the germs house to small brother, mother, and father. It appeared that four of these were with something that the whole winter.

The infant was colicky. From the spring, following a household bout with influenza, Lisa's friend supplied the title of a behavioral therapist who she explained could have the ability to shed some light about the recurrent diseases of Lisa's small boys. In the first consultation, Lisa declared the previous four decades of her household's lifestyle, culminating at current influenza where the small boys were recuperating. They were exhausted, tired, not sleeping well, and usually under sunlight. With summer vacation just around the corner, Lisa had been distressed to receive her family back on the right track.

The words of this nutritionist proved rather easy: Start feeding your household foods which are fresh and ready in your home. Start buying fruits and veggies, and make some simple recipes using rice and other grains. Learn how to create healthy and wholesome dishes to your loved ones. These phrases triggered Lisa to remember when she had been a kid about the time of her very own small boys. She remembered her mother fixing large fruit salads using lemon. She recalled delicious dishes of homemade soup along with hot fresh bread. At the instant, Lisa knew what she needed to make happen for her boys. And she'd make it occur. Approximately six months after, we received a telephone call from Lisa. I can hear the grin brimming in her voice. "You cannot think the shift in our loved ones. Ricky has had just one cold in the previous six weeks, and we are all sleeping much better, and also the infant is happy and sleeping soundly during the night. Four days per week, we have a family walk after breakfast or after dinner. And guess what? I have lost thirty-five lbs., and that I was not dieting! I'm better than I have ever felt."

Giving Forth

Forgiveness is a significant step in enjoying yourself. At any time, you forgive, you're "committing forth" or "letting go" of a thing you're holding inside you. Let's be clear about this: bias is simply for you, not anybody else. It's not a kind of accepting, condoning, or justifying somebody else's activities. It's a practice of letting go of an adverse impression that has remained within you too long. It's the letting go of any emotion or idea which can be an obstacle between you and enjoying yourself and getting what you desire.

A lot of us are considerably more crucial and much tougher on ourselves than we're on the others. When you continue to notions of what you should or should not have completed, you're not enjoying yourself. Instead, you're putting alert energy to negative beliefs about yourself. Ideas like "I should have obtained a stroll " or even "I shouldn't have eaten this second slice of pie" can also be regarded as self-punishing. Sometimes, penalizing yourself, either by lack of overeating or eating, may even lead to discount for your wellbeing. By shifting your focus to self-appreciation, you go from the negative to the positive, that is quite a bit more conducive to self-loving.

CHAPTER 10:

Breathing Exercises

Types of Breathing Exercises

1. Sama Vritti or "Equivalent Breathing"

Sama Vritti Pranayama is an incredible unwinding instrument that can help clear your psyche, loosen up your body, and enable you to center. You can do it anywhere. Simply locate an agreeable seat with your back upheld and feet on the floor. Put shortly viewing your normal breath. Without transforming anything, watch the common inward breath, the exhalation and the regular stops between every breath.

After a couple of rounds, you could take the tally up to 6, yet you can remain at 4 or on the off chance that you discover you are battling with the breath just lower it to 2 or 3 until it feels simpler. Attempt to develop a similar nature of breath toward the start, center, and end of the tally.

The breath ought not to be constrained or stressed during Pranayama.

Level of difficulty: Beginner

2. Stomach Breathing Technique

Diaphragmatic breathing is a sort of a breathing activity that fortifies your stomach, a significant muscle that causes you to relax. This breathing activity is additionally here and there called paunch breathing or stomach breathing. One of the greatest advantages of diaphragmatic breathing is lessening stress. The most fundamental kind of diaphragmatic breathing is finished by breathing in through your nose and breathing out through your mouth.

Level of difficulty: Beginner

3. Nadi Shodhana or "Substitute Nostril Breathing"

Nadi signifies "channel," and Shodhana signifies "purging" or "purifying."The Nadi Shodhana Pranayama will loosen up the brain and set it up for reflection, making it an incredible procedure to perform before ruminating. It can likewise be polished as a major aspect of the Padma Sadhana sequence. Alternate nostril breathing can be valuable for both the start and prepared yoga expert.

Level of difficulty: Intermediate

4. Kapalabhati or "Skull Shining Breath"

Kapalabhati is a middle of the road to-cutting edge pranayama that comprises of short, groundbreaking breathes out and latent breathes in. This activity is a customary inner sanitization practice, or Kriya, that tone and purges the respiratory framework by empowering the arrival of poisons and waste issues. It goes about as a tonic for the framework, reviving and restoring the body and psyche. "Kapala" signifies the skull and "bhati" signifies light.

Level of difficulty: Advanced

5. Dynamic Relaxation

A dynamic Relaxation is an approach, which enables you to stay loose and alert while performing ordinary undertakings and meeting the physical and mental requests of day by day life. It is not just pertinent to recuperation from sickness, incapacity, and constant issue yet additionally to expand potential. Dynamic Relaxation utilizes appendage developments to prepare the mind and cerebrum movement to prepare the non-useful appendages at the same time, along these lines quickening progress and advantages with fewer exercise reiterations.

Level of difficulty: Beginner

6. Guided Visualization

Symbolism is unfathomably easy to utilize. You should simply tune in to your guide while they lead you through a progression of unwinding visualizations. Guided perceptions are generally custom fitted to enable you to achieve explicit objectives, from donning accomplishments to physical recuperating, to individual change, or profound unwinding.

At the point when utilized accurately, these representations are distinctive to the point that they really realize quantifiable positive changes in both your body and psyche.

Guided representation and guided reflection are utilized from various perspectives, from restorative treatment that upgrades mending to profound unwinding. Practically any part of one's life can be improved by the utilization of positive symbolism.

Level of difficulty: Intermediate

Mindful Meditation

Care is presently being inspected logically and has been seen as a key component in stress decrease and generally speaking satisfaction. Most religions incorporate some kind of petition or reflection method that helps move your contemplations from your typical distractions toward a valuation for the minute and a bigger point of view on life. However, its underlying foundations start from Buddhism.

Careful contemplation is an incredible method to expand the center, decline pressure, and invigorate your creativity. Learning how to do careful reflection takes some time and practice, however, you can show yourself how to do it. You can likewise figure out how to join care methods into your regular day to day existence, for example, when you are eating, strolling, or approaching your other everyday errands.

Here are the means by which you do it:

When you have your seat and your spot, feel free to plunk down. Take a stance that is upstanding yet not inflexible. The thought is to take a stance that mirrors your natural splendid mental stability, so one that is honorable yet not firm. The back is forthright with the bend in the lower back that is normally there.

You might need to begin with only a five to 10-moment reflection and work up from that point. Try not to begin ruminating for an hour, as this can appear to be overpowering. Rather, pick little additions of time to focus on, and on the off chance that you need, increment the time.

The second piece of the training is working with the breath. In this training rest your consideration daintily (indeed, gently) on the breath. Feel it as it comes into your body and as it goes out. There is no uncommon method to take in this system. By and by, we are keen on how we as of now are, not how we are in the event that we control our breath. In the event that you find that you are, actually, controlling your breath somehow or another, simply given it a chance to be that way.

It might take you a smidgen of time to settle in and start to confine from every one of the things going on in your life. Particularly in the event that you have had a distressing day, you may end up considering what occurred or about things that need to occur later on. You may feel your feelings mixing. The majority of this is all right. Notice that your brain is moving, and let it move for a piece as you settle in. At the point when you see that you have gotten so made up for the lost time in musings that you have overlooked that you're sitting in the room, just delicately take yourself back to the breath.

At last, and maybe above all, recall that care reflection is tied in with working on being aware of whatever occurs. As you reflect, advise yourself that you have command over what contemplations and feelings your lock-in.

1. Relax!

You are continually breathing, yet how frequently would you say you are mindful of it? Broaden your sitting practice into monitoring your breath while at work, home or while doing diverse day by day errands. Know about your breath in the staple line, when anticipating a guest, in-car influxes, previously or after dinners.

2. Appreciate the Silence

Our lives are definitely not calm. At the point when it isn't the sound of traffic, planes above, collaborators or individual understudies babbling hectically, or the ping of a telephone call or message, it's the music or program we put on to fill the void.

Set aside the effort to investigate calm. You'll discover that quiet is rarely quiet – even in the remotest of zones there's wind, leaves stirring, birdsong and creature clamors, downpour falling, etc.

Utilize the sounds that rise up out of the calm as a major aspect of your mindfulness practice. Tenderly investigate sentiments of nervousness that may emerge when you do without the typical interruptions, at that point let them proceed to come back to the artistic work of careful tuning in.

3. Go for a Nice Stroll

Locate an intriguing spot to walk and put in no time flat in the consciousness of each progression. Focus on the weight of your feet as they clean the ground and lift up once more. Notice how the muscles in your toes and legs work to drive your body forward. On the off chance that you can, make a strolling reflection part of your customary practice.

4. Stop being a Busy-Body

See what happens when you quit performing various tasks, even quickly. Work on one errand or undertaking before proceeding onward to the following with the goal that each task profits by your complete consideration. Figure out how to concentrate on one errand whether it is eating, resurfacing furniture or composing a significant discourse.

Because of your customary care work on (accepting you do as such), it will be simpler for you to see when your musings have meandered. Bring them back, tenderly however immovably, similarly as you do when you contemplate, and keep giving your full focus to the job needing to be done.

5. Tasks! Tasks! Tasks!

As you approach your family unit tasks, empty yourself into them wholeheartedly. Not exclusively will you end up with a cleaner restroom, progressively sorted out the carport and smirch free windows, you will likewise encounter a decent arrangement of appreciation. As you walk, eat, travel and by and large continue on ahead, make sure to take care, appreciation and liberality part of your experience. At suppers, be aware of what you are eating – the nourishment on the fork, however everything that went into getting that feast on your plate in any case.

CHAPTER 11:

Eat Healthy and Sleep Better with Hypnosis

Make yourself comfortable. Find the perfect sleep position. Inhale through your nose and exhale through your mouth.

Again, inhale through your nose and this time as you exhale close your eyes.

Repeat this one more time and relax.

Sharpen your breathing focus.

Find stillness in every breath you take, relieve yourself from any tension and relax.

Let your body relax, soften your heart, quiet your anxious mind and open to whatever you experience without fighting.

Simply allow your thoughts and experiences to come and go without grasping at them.

Reduce any stress, anxiety, or negative emotions you might have, cool down become deeply and comfortably relaxed.

That's fine.

And as you continue to relax then you can begin the process of reprogramming your mind for your weight loss success because with the right mindset, then you can think positively about what you want to achieve. It begins with changing your mindset and attitude, because the key to losing weight all starts in the mind. One of the very first things you must throw out the window (figuratively) before you start your journey to weight loss is negativity. Negative thinking will just lead you nowhere. It will only pull your moods down which might trigger emotional eating. Thus, you'll eat more, adding up to that unwanted weight instead of losing it. Remember that you must need to break your old bad habits and one of them is negative self-talk. You need to change your negative mental views and turn them into positive ones. For example, instead of telling yourself after a few days of workout that nothing is happening or changing, tell yourself that you have done a set of physical activities you have never imagine you can or will do. Make it a point to pat yourself on the back for every little progress you make every day, may it be five additional crunches from what you did yesterday. Understand and accept that this process is a complete transformation, a metamorphosis if you will. This understanding is going to make the process smoother, and less painful.

Aside from being positive, you should also be realistic. Don't expect an immediate change in your body. Keep in mind that losing weight is not an overnight thing. It is a long-term process and gradual progress. Set and focus on your goals to keep that negativity at bay. Losing weight needs consistent reminders and focus on proper mental preparations. Always keep yourself motivated. Train yourself to think positive all the time.

Don't compare yourself to others, because it will not help you attain your goals in losing weight. First and foremost, keep in mind that each one of us has different body types and compositions. There is a certain diet that may work on you, but not so much for the others. Possibly, some people might need more carbohydrates in their diet, while you might need to drop that and add more protein in your meals. Each one of us is unique. Therefore, your diet plan will surely differ from the person next to you.

Comparing yourself to other people's progress is just a negative thought and will just be unhelpful to you. Remember, always keep a positive outlook and commit to it before you start your diet. For the sake of your long-term success, leave the comparison trap. You're not exactly like the people you idolize and they're not exactly like you and that's perfectly fine. Accept that, embrace that and move on with your personal goals.

Be realistic in setting your goals. Think about small and easy to achieve goals that will guide you towards a long term of healthy lifestyle changes. Your goals should be healthy for your body. If you want to truly lose weight and keep it off, it will be a slow uphill battle, with occasional dips and times you'll want to quit. If you expect progress too fast, you will eventually not be able to reach your goals and become discouraged. Don't add extra obstacles for yourself, plan your goals carefully.

If possible, try to find someone who has similar goals as you and work on them together. Two is always better than one, and having someone who understands what you are undergoing can be such a relief! An added benefit of having a partner-in-crime (or several) is that you can always hold each other accountable. Accountability is one thing that is easy to start being lax after the first few weeks of a new weight loss program, especially if results aren't quite where you want them to be.

Write down a realistic timetable that you can follow. Start a journal about your daily exercises and meal plan. You can cross out things that you have done already or add new ones along the way. Plot your physical activities. Make time and mark your calendar with daily physical activities. Try to incorporate at least a 15-minute workout on your busy days.

When you become aware of a thought or belief that pins the blame for your extra weight on something outside yourself, if you can find examples of people who've overcome that same cause, realize that it's decision time for you. Choose for yourself whether this is a thought you want to embrace and accept. Does this thought support you living your best life? Does it move you toward your goals, or does it give you an excuse not to go after them?

If you determine your thought no longer serves you, you get to choose another thought instead. Instead of pointing to some external, all-powerful cause for you being overweight, you can choose something different. Track your progress by writing down your step count or workouts daily to keep track of your progress.

Celebrate and embrace your results. Since the path to a healthy lifestyle is mostly hard work and discipline, try to reward yourself for every progress even if it is small. Treat yourself for a day of pampering, travel to a place you have been wanting to visit, go hiking, have a movie date with friends or get a new pair of shoes. These kinds of rewards provide you gratification and accomplishments that will make you keep going. Little things do count and little things also deserve recognition. But keep in mind that your rewards should not compromise your diet plan.

You can also do something like joining an athletic event, a fun run, where you can meet new people that share the same ideals of a healthy lifestyle. You get to learn more about weight loss from others and also share your knowledge. You need to find a source of motivation and keep that source of motivation fresh in your mind so you don't forget why you embarked on this journey to begin with.

As you focus on your journey of weight loss, keep your stress at bay because too much stress is harmful for the body in many ways, but it also can cause people to gain weight. When the body is under stress, the body will automatically release many hormones and among one of them is cortisol. When the body is under duress and stress, cortisol is released, is can ignite the metabolism, for a period of time. However, if the body remains in stressful conditions, the hormone cortisol will continue to be released, and actually slow down the metabolism resulting in weight gain.

Everyone experiences stress; there is just no getting around that fact. However, minimizing stressors, as well as learning how to manage the stress in your life will not only help you with you with losing weight, but it will also make a more attractive you! High stress in anyone's life often brings out the worst in people. When you are trying to get a man, you want them to see the best of you, not the stressed out you. While you are decreasing your stress level, you will want to increase the amount of sleep you get each night. Lack of sleep is a link to weight gain and because of this, ensuring adequate and appropriate sleep is crucial when trying to lose weight. Sleep is vital for the wellbeing of the body, and the ability for the mind to function, but it is also related to maintaining weight. If you are tired, make sure you sleep, rest or relax, so you are not prone to gaining weight. When a person gets more sleep, the hormone leptin will rise and when this happens the appetite decreases which will also decrease body weight.

Gratitude is important in this journey because it teaches you how to make peace with your body, no matter what shape, size or weight it has at the moment. It makes you look at your body with full acceptance and love, saying: "I'm grateful for my body the way it is." It stops you from beating yourself up for being overweight, unhealthy or out of shape. Be grateful for this learning experience, accept yourself the way you are, and take massive action to get your balance back.

When you express gratitude, you vibrate on a higher energy level, you are positive and happy, and you are simply in the state of satisfaction.

The more things you can find to be grateful for during your weight loss journey, the easier it will be to maintain a positive attitude and keep your motivation up.

It will also get you past those tough moments when you are feeling demotivated to take action and stick to the exercising or eating plan.

This means that you start expressing gratitude for the aspects of your body you would like to have, as if you already have them now. Be grateful for your sexy legs and slim waist. Be grateful for your increased energy levels and strength. Be grateful for the ability to wear smaller clothes. You get the drill. Feel the positive energy of gratitude flowing through your body as you imagine these things are true. By going through this exercise you'll notice the positive change in your thought patterns.

CHAPTER 12:

Common Fitness Misconceptions

The world of fitness is full of persuasive theories that claim that it will assist you to accomplish your objectives. Some are valuable, while others may take you down a street of unnecessary hard work and misleading outcomes. This section tackles the very well-known misconceptions when utilizing training and nutrition to attain your physique.

Misconception #1: Cardio to Shed Weight

You frequently see folks running plenty of miles on the treadmill in hopes of slimming down. Though cardio enhances general wellbeing, it's not essential to be able to burn off fat. Cardio exercises like jogging, biking, and the elliptical machines are tools to help rapid weight reduction, but the determining factor to if your weight changes is the body's balance of calories. Cardio may be a waste of time if your diet is not in check. By way of instance, somebody may run 10 mph that burns off 1,000 calories, then consume 1,500 calories and lead to gaining weight. Weight reduction is best accomplished by controlling your diet plan. A banana is usually 100 calories, and it requires about 100 calories to run 1 mile. So, could it be simpler to run a mile or just not eat a banana? Unless you are a fighter and fantasize over bananas, then it would probably be simpler to prevent running a mile. This is a prime case of becoming smarter about attaining your target, rather than overworking yourself.

Once your diet is in check, you can then contemplate aerobic to Burn calories. While cardio encourages weight reduction, doing too much can often pose a level look on your muscles. Weight training, on the other hand, develops your muscles, which adds additional detail to your body. Utilize your calories to the exercises which will develop the type of results you desire. Even though you can get a fantastic body without using cardio, it's beneficial under certain circumstances. It may be quite a challenge to give your body sufficient nourishment while adhering to a low-carb diet. Consequently, cardio is helpful for burning extra calories, which can enable you to refrain from reducing the number of calories you eat while attempting to eliminate fat.

Misconception #2: Toning

To be able to obtain a "toned" look that many people need, an individual should either reduce their body fat or build additional muscle. By doing this, you are able to specify your body even faster. You may just make your muscles bigger or smaller, and you may only gain or eliminate fat. Fat can't turn into muscle building, nor will muscle turn into fat. Decreasing your own body fat percentage needs, you to burn off more calories than you eat. To be able to construct muscle, you need to challenge your muscles enough to develop via the use of workout. Some people frequently want to remain the identical weight whilst attaining a toned body. As a pound of muscle is denser than a pound of fat, then it's likely to get a more defined body when weighing the same. Muscles require a good deal longer to develop than required to eliminate fat. Thus, your weight will probably decrease because of the reduction of fat when reaching these outcomes in a brief time period.

Misconception #3: Targeting Fat Loss

Some people want to shed fat just in their gut, legs, or another portion of the body. Targeting the decrease in fat in a particular place in your body isn't feasible. The regions where you lose and gain fat are already given by your genetics. A few areas of fat on the body will take longer to go away than many others. By way of instance, someone may lose the majority of the fat in their arms while still holding a great deal of fat around their belly. The decrease in belly is common among the more challenging regions to eliminate fat. To be able to burn off fat in that stubborn region, you may only need to keep exercising. Finally, the body will choose to burn off fat from the stubborn regions once it reaches a lower proportion of body fat loss. There isn't any exercise or material which will make it possible for you to burn off fat in one particular region of the body.

Misconception #4: Ab-Training

Some People Today believe that in order to possess great abs, you need to educate them hard daily. The abdominal muscles need time to recuperate exactly like other muscles on the entire body, so educating them regular is not vital. Abs best react to high repetitions and brief rest periods between sets. Implementing extra weight on your ab training can help develop greater mass. Make sure that you select exercises which will target every section of their abdominals such as the upper, lower, and oblique locations. It's crucial to not forget that your body fat percent has to be low enough to determine your abs. You are able to train your abs sufficient to develop, but in case you've got a thick layer of fat within the stomach, then they won't be observable.

Misconception #5: Eating Junk Food

Eating junk food does not need to get in the method of attaining Your exercise target. The more you understand the way your body handles food, is that the guilt you'll feel about everything you eat. Whatever you eat or drink will probably be simplified to a carbs, fat, or protein. Thus, even in the event that you eat a cheeseburger, however, you're still inside your macronutrient targets for the day, then you won't disrupt the improvement of losing weight or building muscle.

Together with the IIFYM (If It Fits Your Macros) procedure for shedding weight, we often get confused into believing you ought to eat as much junk food that you need so long as it fits into your macronutrient objectives. Despite the fact that doing so can permit you to realize your desired body, your inner health will be in danger. Before committing yourself to a cheeseburger or milkshake, make confident you are getting the majority of your nutrition from whole foods every day.

Misconception #6: Alcohol

Most individuals are afraid to drink alcoholic drinks in panic. It will ruin the advancement towards their exercise goal. It's fine to get some alcohol so long as it's in moderation. Alcohol has calories (7 calories per gram), therefore understanding the amount from the beverage and the number of calories you're permitted can help you keep on pace for achieving your exercise goal. It's possible to substitute the calories out of drinking to get some fat or carbohydrates on this day, yet make certain that you're getting enough wholesome nourishment from food because alcohol won't supply any. Implementing aerobic or additional physical activity on your program might help burn extra calories to permit space for a beverage or 2. It's helpful to consume a lot of water ahead to reduce dehydration and extra drinking. Possessing an occasional beer or wine won't mess up your advancement so long as you can fit it into a wholesome diet.

Misconception #7: Too Much Sugar

It's true that consuming much sugar can result in long-term health risks like diabetes, organ failure, and lots of ailments. However, concerning fat loss, eating considerable quantities of sugar won't keep you from losing weight provided that the essential calories to burn off fat are fulfilled over time. All carbohydrates are broken down into sugar once digested from the human body. Some food resources like complex carbohydrates take longer to break down, while some happen to be in a very simple form such as sugar. Because your entire body uses carbohydrates as a key source of fuel during physical action, the more active you're is that, the more carbohydrates you're allowed. Those who burn a lot of calories may eliminate consuming more sugar as it's being used rather than accumulating in the human body.

Sugar has a bad rap as it's easy to overeat. Just as Whatever else, having a lot of anything could be bad for you. Consuming whole foods, that can be more filling and nutritious, helps to modulate the general usage of sugar. Concerning losing weight, substituting sweet foods like raw honey or agave nectar for pure sugar is insignificant because they still comprise simple carbohydrates which break down to sugar on your system. Sweeteners like 'Equal', ''Splenda', or stevia will nevertheless make a difference because they include zero calories. Recognizing how many carbohydrates You're permitted Can allow you to be aware of how much sugar you can consume while pursuing Your exercise target.

Misconception #8: Too Much Sodium

Prioritizing your salt consumption plays an insignificant role in burning building or fat muscle. This is much more of a precaution into your overall wellbeing rather than a requirement for building a fantastic physique. Regulating amounts of sodium may reduce blood pressure while reducing the dangers of cardiovascular disease and stroke.

When sodium is in the human body, it complies with water and keeps the Equilibrium of fluids. Additionally, it works with potassium to maintain electric procedures across cell membranes, and this can be essential for neural transmission, muscle contraction, and other functions. The body can't work without sodium, therefore restricting your consumption with no respect to just how much you truly desire, may be a possible risk.

An increase in sodium induces your system to consume more water, which is why your body weight changes throughout the day. Reducing sodium intake will help to decrease body fat but is largely due to the temporary reduction of water. It's necessary to remember that in most instances, the objective isn't to eliminate water except to burn off fat. There are significant instances to monitor sodium intake, for example, if preparing for a bodybuilding contest or photoshoot. Bodybuilders or versions may control their salt consumption to present their body a sterile, skin-tight allure when they're already lean enough to observe the detail of the muscles.

Misconception #9: Metabolism

Individuals often use their metabolism as a justification for why they have not attained their physical fitness goals. Other people assert that ingesting particular foods can improve their metabolism and lead them to drop weight. Since the expression metabolism finds its way to misleading notions every day, it's a "grey" area for the majority of people and may use some caution. Metabolism is how much food that your body can process every day. It's the procedure by which your body transforms what you eat and drink into energy your body can utilize. The rate of your metabolism or basal metabolic rate (BMR) determines the number of calories your body will need so as to operate. A number of things that affect your BMR comprise your own body size, gender, and age.

For the most part, your own body's energy requirement to procedure food remains relatively steady and is not readily changed5. Thus, it's immaterial to rely on particular foods to improve your metabolism to be able to eliminate weight. Your body was created for you to meet the number of calories necessary to encourage your metabolism by simply telling you that you are hungry once you want more calories and to stop eating once you have sufficient calories.

CHAPTER 13:

All-Natural Ways to Burn Fats

You do not need to invest thousands of dollars on the market's best fat heater to melt excess fats because you can burn fats naturally. Remember that this should be done with appropriate exercise along with a healthy and balanced diet if you want to discover how to burn tummy fat quickly for men. Keep in mind that you will certainly not have the ability to do this by focusing on a healthy diet or regular exercise alone. Another thing that you need to keep in mind is that losing stubborn belly fats could be impossible if you are to focus on a specific area alone. Right here are some techniques on how you can do it:

- Reduce your caloric consumption:

Reduce the section dimensions of your meals. It is essential to consume reasonably and not as high as you want for you to eat fewer calories. The suggestion is that you should consume fewer calories than you shed. The lesser the number of calories you take, the much better. Perhaps replacing heavy meals with vegetables and fruits will certainly do the trick.

Counting calories is another essential action man need to take. You can figure out how much food you can eat and how much you got to work out. Some men count calories, but they do not count the two to three beers they have in the evening, which is truly bad. Everything that goes right into your mouth needs to be noted.

- Eating Healthy

Learning how to burn belly fat quickly for men ought to include a healthy and balanced diet plan. Bear in mind that eating fast food, way too much coffee, and tea, soft drinks, and dealing with unneeded anxiety from school or work can only add up to your weight gain.

What you must find are the foods that can help you burn fats. Make sure you find out how to integrate healthy foods into your diet, and also, this ought to include foods such as vegetables and even fruits, lean meat, whole-grain grains, and beans, to name a few.

- Eat foods rich in fiber.

Fiber, as you know, is extremely useful in washing out contaminants, excess fats, and other unwanted bits in your body. You can eat a lot of vegetables and fruits day-to-day, and you can also consume alcohol lots of water. And if you can, get involved in the habit of drinking green tea. Green tea contains antioxidants and other compounds that help burn fats naturally.

- Increase your physical activity:

It is recommended to have three to five times weekly exercise regimen to lose weight. It should be that the exercise is at a moderate intensity to attain physical changes on your body. If you opt for a more vigorous aerobic activity, the better it is. When you don't have time to go to an aerobics class or enroll in a gym, that is where the problem lies. To solve this, you just need to convert your everyday activities into a more active one. For example, replace your hobby of riding on an elevator with climbing on the stairs, walking to the office instead of riding on a car. There could be too much, and you just need to be creative on your exercise plan.

Fat loss for men is even more natural than it is for ladies. If a man just has a couple of pounds that they would like to lose, they can generally shed it rapidly.

What might take a woman a couple of months to lose, a man can do it in a few weeks. Their bodies are just rigged in different ways, and they can do this, whether it's reasonable or otherwise. What are a few of the more crucial things you'll need to bear in mind to drop weight? One of the main formulae is exercise

Exercising regularly is an indispensable part of the process of weight-loss. Lifting weights is a great thing to obtain included within weight loss for men. They will, in turn, burn more calories when you train your muscle mass. They will be burning calories also while you're sleeping. This means that you will reduce weight quicker.

- Limit Insulin Release

Insulin is a storage hormone, and it can be lessened by removing unexpected dives in blood glucose. This is done only by eating more frequently. Primarily what you do is that you fuel your body much more equally throughout the day, and for that reason, your sugar degrees will be steadier. Snacks are essential and vital as they will help you to decrease blood insulin launch. In enhancement, you should drink more water, when feasible with lemon in it (or a few other citric juices).

- Be positive and live a stress-free life.

Sometimes, problems can add to your weight challenge. You will want to eat more if you get depressed. So, to avoid getting yourself into this situation, surround yourself with happy people in a healthy environment.

The Fat Burning Furnace Reviewed

There are fat heaters available for men only, these unique formulas for men increase the testosterone level, thus boosting the fat loss process. They are specifically created to include many different active ingredients that are secure for men who prefer to reduce weight, melt fat, and improve muscle-building initiatives.

A common component in testosterone-based fat burners is high levels of caffeine.

L-Glutamine assists the muscles to recover after a man has completed his workout. Taken into consideration that reducing weight is a mixture of diet, exercise, and making use of fat burners having L-glutamine in this supplement improves its use because it also aids the immune system.

Lastly, cinnamon is contained in this fat burning supplement because it enhances the metabolic rate and diminishes the risks of diabetic issues.

A testosterone booster in the nutritional supplement of a man is always a great way to construct and melt the fat muscle mass too. L-Arginine is one more healthy protein item that expands the capillary, enabling more oxygen as well as nutrients to go into the bloodstream, inevitably enhancing the muscular tissues of a person.

You can choose from several fat burners for men available in the market; for instance, the ones pointed out over or any type of variety of combinations.

What about the ingredients type?

If not, do not take possibilities. Keep in mind any adverse effects related to the ingredients and take just the recommended dose.

Each of those items has various active ingredients and formulas. Nonetheless, some are better for men because they are targeted at not just the breakdown as well as the burning of the fat, but they are also aimed at bodybuilding. For your study, there are many organic food shops and even websites that specifically offer a selection of fat burners created for men.

Depending on the weight management requirements you want, and the current state of your health, your option of the fat burner needs not to be challenging to discover. But make sure that you include exercise in your strategy for weight reduction.

The truth is that men benefit nicely from programs like the Fat Burning Furnace. That's because as soon as they start, they begin to appreciate it. Before they understand it, the metabolic rate in their bodies has gotten much more energetic, and the weight simply starts to thaw off them permanently.

What happens is, as the people begin to do the regimens for twenty minutes a day and three days per week, they don't recognize that they have started to acquire a much leaner muscular tissue. And as that happens, the heating system is fueled, causing the fat to melt away simply.

You can prepare on shedding a great deal of body fat and get a lot of lean muscle mass. Not the big large muscles that men frequently link with the muscle contractors and body home builders.

While it may be helpful for you is you have a fitness center membership where you can use some professional equipment to help you along your journey, it is not a compulsory requirement but will produce the wanted results. A collection of dumbbells is one of the many things that will help you along your course to the goal and well worth the small investment if you don't already have some.

Similar to any routine that entails physical tasks, you must make sure that you are physically fit to do the procedures that will be needed. If you have a physical limitation that would prevent you from exercise or if you have particular troubles that need food policy, such as diabetes mellitus, you might want to get your doctor's approval before you begin.

If you want to learn how to burn belly fat fast for men, remember that this should be done with proper exercise along with a healthy diet.

CHAPTER 14:

Overcoming Negative Habits

Fortunately, most of our days have a sort of "groove." Actions in a plan that you perform with little thought are performed almost automatically. Otherwise, our lives become tediously complicated, and we spend a lot of time figuring out how to tie our shoes, prepare our meals, go to work, and more. In this way, we can carry out our daily routines with almost no thought and focus our attention on more demanding activities. Repetitive work in life becomes a habit.

Habits can also be undesirable, and these grooves are deeply rooted in today's patterns. They are against us because they waste our time. For example, if you know that you have a limited amount of time to get to work after waking up in the morning, you'll notice that in the middle of breakfast you'll find the morning paper at the table, pick it up, and usually spend the next hour studying. Spend In the daily news, you could spend a good deal of the rest of your time explaining delays or looking for new jobs.

By the way, in our discussion of habits, we call them "desired" or "undesired" rather than "good" or "bad." The words "good" and "bad" have moral implications. These mean certain decisions. In the example cited in the paragraph above, reading a newspaper is not morally "bad," but not desirable at this time.

The terms "desired" and "undesirable" are the terms "ego," meaning self-determination, not decisions made externally. As with psychoanalysis, our goal is to push material from the "conscience" camp into the "ego" realm.

Such habits have physical-neurologic-foundation. The neural pathways in our body can be compared to unpaved roads. This road is smooth before vehicles drive on dirt roads. When a car first rides on the road, its tires leave marks, but the ruts are flat. Rain and wind can easily pass by and smooth the road again. However, after 100 rides with deeper and deeper tires, rain and wind make little impression on the deep ruts. They stay there.

The same applies to people. To expand the metaphor a little, we were born with a smooth street in our heads. When a young child first buttons a jacket or ties a shoe, the effort is tedious, clumsy, and frustrating. More trials are needed until the child gets the hang of it, and a successful move becomes a behavioral pattern.

From a physiological point of view, these movement instructions travel along nerve paths to the muscles and back again. The message is sent to the central nervous system along an afferent pathway. The "I want to lift my legs" impulse continues in the efferent pathway from the central nervous system to my muscles: "Raise my legs." After a while, such messages are automatically enriched by countless repetitions and automatically sent at electrical speed.

Return to the car and the street. Suppose the car decides to avoid a worn groove and take a new path. What's going on the car will go straight back into the old ditch. Like people trying to get out of old habits, they tend to revert to old habits.

Still, we haven't developed any unwanted habits. We learn them, and we can rewind the learning. It can be unconditional. And here, self-hypnosis takes place, pushing the individual out of the established habit gap in a smooth manner of new behavior.

The advantage it offers compared to simple willpower trial and error results from an increase in the state of consciousness that characterizes the state of self-hypnosis. As a neurological phenomenon in itself, this elevated state of consciousness appears to elevate the individual over previous behavioral patterns. A further extension of the unpaved road analogy is that the hovercraft slides a few centimeters above the road, over a rut or habit. Regardless of the habit of working, the implementation process is the same. Only the verbal implant and the image below are different. To encapsulate the induction process, count one, for one thing, two for two things and count three for three things:

1. Please raise your eyes as high as possible.

2. Still staring, slowly close your eyes and take a deep breath.

3. Exhale, relax your eyes, and float your body. Then, if time permits, spend a little more time and introduce yourself to the most comfortable, calm, and pleasant place in your imagination.

Now, when you float deep inside the resting chair, you will feel a little away from your body. It's another matter, so you can give her instructions on how to behave.

At this point, the specific purpose of self-hypnosis determines the expression and image content of the syllogism. It provides suggestions for discussing different habits that can be followed as shown or modified as needed. This strategy can help overcome the habit of overeating.

Overall, we are a country boasting abundant food. Most of us (with the blatant and lamentable exception) have enough money to make sure we are comfortably overeating. As a result, many of us get obese. So, the weight loss business is a big industry. Tablet makers, diet developers, and exercise studios will not confuse customers who want to lose weight.

It is said that every fat person who has a hard time escaping has lost weight. Unfortunately, too often, the lean man spends his life, nevertheless never succeeding in his escape. Despite the image of a funny fat man, everyone rarely enjoys being overweight-most people become unhappy, rarely so confident, and less than confident and ruining their lives. Obesity seems to creep on only some of us, and by the time we notice it, it is a painful habit to overeat or eat, like the excess weight itself.

Self-hypnosis can help this lean man release his bond of "too hard" and start a new life. An article in the International Journal of Clinical and Experimental Hypnosis (January 1975) reports on such cases. Sidney E. and Mitchell P. Pulver cite family doctors study hypnosis in medical and dental practice.

Dr. Roger Bernhardt, while mentioning one of his overweight patients, said that "I brought the patient to the hospital for about a year and a half ago. She went to many doctors to cut back. She said she was rarely leaving home because she was extremely obese; she was relaxing and avoiding people. She came in for £ 380. I started trans in my first session. She continued on a diet and focused on telling her she would like people when she lost weight. She came for the first three or four sessions each week, after which I started teaching her self-hypnosis. Now, this woman lost a total of £ 150, but beyond that, she became another person. She was virtually introverted and rarely came out of her home. She dared to do a part-time job in cosmetics. She hosts a party to show off her cosmetics and hypnotizes herself before the party. She became the state's second-largest saleswoman and earned tens of thousands of dollars."

Simply put, here are the therapies you should use when using self-hypnosis for weight management. After provoking self-hypnosis, mentally recite the syllogism. "I need my body alive. To the extent I want to live, I protect my body just as I protect it."

In the case of a tie mate picture, one can imagine himself in two situations where he is likely to overeat: between meals and at the dining table. With his eyes closed, he imagines a movie screen on the wall. He is on the screen himself, in every situation he finds when he is reading, chatting with others, watching TV, or having trouble calorie counting.

Instead of reaching for popcorn, potato chips, or peanuts as before, he is now simply focusing on the conversation, the television screen, or the printed page, perhaps except for a glass of water, and I congratulate you on being unfamiliar with anything at the table. The second scene that catches your eye is the dining table. Do you tend to grab this second loaf? Instead, put your hand on your forehead and remember, "Protect my body." Looking at a cake, a loaf, a potato, or a cake raises the idea, "This is for someone. I'm good enough". With the fork down, take a deep breath and be proud to help one-person flow through the body. Then, imagine a very simple and effective exercise method that simply puts your hand on the edge of the table and pushes it. Better yet, stand up from the chair and leave the table at this point.

Here's another image I'd recommend to a self-hypnotist. If you introduce yourself to the screen of this fictional movie, you will find yourself slim. Give yourself the ideal line that you want to see to others. Cut the abdomen and waistline to the desired ratio. Take an imaginary black pencil, sketch the entire picture, and make the lines sharp and solid. Hold photo Because you can keep this slender picture, you can lose weight. Then get out of your hypnosis and repeat it regularly every few hours. Exercise is especially useful during the temptation to be used as a comfortable, calorie-free substitute for fatty snacks or as an additional serving with meals. It would be a good time to practice it just before dinner.

As a complement to this discussion, Dr. Roger Bernhardt, while talking about a patient, wrote:" I would like to touch on one of my patients, Mr. Happiness. (He often said to me, so he has this name in my reasoning: "All I want from life is being happy.")

Happiness and I have had many problems together, including my sister's suicide, a heart attack, the end of his previous business, and the establishment of a new business. But now I'm glad to say; he's a happy retired man. He says he comes every 6 to 8 weeks, "to keep the wheels oiled."

Shortly after becoming familiar with hypnosis, I enthusiastically talked to him about it and invited him to use it to treat current problems. He refused. He was afraid of that. After a while, I wrote a small brochure about hypnosis. One day, I handed a copy to Mr. Happiness. A few weeks later, he said, "Oh, that's funny. It's not psychoanalysis, but he says that all you do is ..." and he repeated the steps of the deployment process. It was

"Yes," I replied, "It's a simple one to two. Do you want to do that?"

Again, he refused: "Oh, not me!"

This issue has not been raised again for several months. It must be mentioned that Mr. Happiness was a fat man and was instructed to lose weight for a heart attack. But what the battle: these potatoes, these rich desserts, and these knives! Then one day, he said to me, "I have done something I recently thought you might be interested in. When I go to bed at night, I count, one, two, three, and I say: I don't eat anything, I just drink grapefruit juice, but I still feel well filled. Patient in the letter: "I only count three.")

CHAPTER 15:

Portion Control Hypnosis

P ortion control tends to be a skill that many people struggle with. Knowing how to eat just enough to help yourself feel satisfied and full, without overeating, can be challenging. This is made even more challenging if you tend to be a stress eater or someone who goes long periods of time without eating and then binge eats. Portion control is an incredibly important element of weight loss as it provides you with the opportunity to get the proper nutrients into your body without overdoing it. As well, if you choose to satisfy one of your cravings or enjoy something more indulgent, portion control enables you to do so without going overboard.

The truth is: most people can eat anything in moderation and not suffer any unwanted consequences from eating that food. For example, if you want to enjoy a piece of brownie with your coffee at the café because you have been craving a brownie, there is typically nothing wrong with doing that. The key is to make sure that you enjoy the brownie, and then you stop. Rather than enjoying that brownie, then eating another piece, then going home and having even more junk food, enjoy that one brownie and then let yourself get back on track with healthy eating. When you can mindfully engage in portion control this way, you can eat just about anything you want without having any problems.

In fact, many famous diets rely more on portion control than anything else because they recognize that portion control is more effective than restricting what people can and cannot eat. The key with portion control is knowing how to actually feel satisfied by your controlled portions, and knowing how to stay committed to them. For many people, this can be challenging. You may feel so happy about eating your brownie or your piece of cake that you want more immediately after. Of course, if you immediately indulge, then you are not effectively engaging in portion control. However, if you instead let yourself enjoy that piece as much as you possibly can and then go back to eating healthy immediately after, then there was no big deal.

Rather than relying solely on portion control as a tool, it is important that you rewire your mind around why you struggle with portion control as it is. Getting to the root cause of your own struggles with portion control, healing your overeating challenges, and rewiring your mind around portion control can be incredibly helpful in allowing you to get what you need out of your diet. This way, rather than dealing with that internal conflict around, "I should stop," you stop naturally because your mind is already wired to stop naturally. As you might suspect, this can be done with subconscious work and hypnosis. However, there are also some conscious-level changes that you should make and things you should become mindful of so that you can navigate portion control both with your conscious mind and your new subconscious habits. This way, you are more likely to be successful with portion control in general.

Why Do People Overeat?

Another reason behind overeating can actually be an eating disorder, which may be caused by underlying conditions such as depression or anxiety, genetics, or other illnesses. If you do have an issue with compulsive overeating and struggle to keep it under control, talking to your doctor is an important way of ruling out possible illness factors that could be contributing to your problems.

When it comes to emotions, everything from stress and anxiety to sadness or discomfort can trigger someone to want to overeat. Believe it or not, the majority of our serotonin and other hormones are produced in the gut. Because of this, when you are feeling stressed out, anxious, sad, or otherwise uncomfortable, you might find yourself craving food. Most people will find themselves craving something specific, such as sweet or salty foods. Other people may find that they are willing to eat whatever is nearby in order to receive that "release" from having something yummy to eat. While overeating due to emotional causes every once in a while, may not necessarily be a bad thing, it is easy for this behavior to turn into a habit. Many people find themselves struggling with overeating due to emotional causes, although stress and sadness tend to be the leading causes of overeating.

Learning how to fix your eating habits by eating more consistently and eating healthier portions at proper meal times is an important way to take care of yourself. Eating regular meals will prevent you from binge eating later on due to being excessively hungry.

Getting to the Root Cause of Your Binge Eating

Understanding your own binge eating habits is important, as this allows you to develop a conscious awareness and a sense of mindfulness around why you are binge eating in the first place. When you are able to understand why you binge eat, resolving the root cause of your binge eating becomes easier because you know what to look for and what to be aware of.

Getting to the root cause of your own binge eating can be done by reflecting on your own binge eating cycles and, if necessary, tracking your binge eating cycles so that you can start to identify any possible patterns that exist around your binge eating behaviors. You can easily do this by keeping a food diary, which is a journal where you log everything you have eaten in a day. Make sure that you write down the time that you ate, what you ate, and how much you ate. Track everything, including little snacks in between. They may not seem significant, but you might be surprised to see how they add up and what comes of those snacks. Often, people find that they are unaware of how problematic their snacking has actually become until they begin to track it.

As you begin looking for the root cause of your binge eating, you might find that there are actually a few root causes. Often, however, most binge eating patterns can be traced back to one "major" root problem that seems to create more problems than the rest. For example, you might find that you have poor eating habits and often find yourself craving low-quality food, but you might realize that this largely stems from you being an emotional eater. Or, you might find that you are an emotional eater because you have poor eating problems and so you realize that, during a moment of stress, eating is one thing you can take care of while everything else might seem out of your control.

It is important that you take the time to identify every single root cause of your binge eating and not just the one that stands out the most. If you are going to have the biggest impact on changing your binge eating patterns, you are going to need to know everything that contributes to your binge eating so that you can be mindful of what might be triggering this behavior. If you do not focus on and heal all of your root causes for binge eating, you might find yourself binge eating out of habit and justifying it by different root causes every single time. The more thorough you can be with healing this, the more effective you will be, too.

With that being said, you may find it to be particularly overwhelming to attempt to actually resolve all of your root causes at once, especially if you have a few. If it does feel overwhelming, you can focus instead on just dealing with the biggest one and then healing one root cause at a time. This way, you can make a significant impact on healing your binge eating problems, but you are still able to remain mindful and aware of your other binge eating triggers.

Learning to Avoid Temptations and Triggers

Once you have a clear understanding of what your binge eating cycles and patterns are like, you can start implementing change to help you avoid temptations and triggers. There are many ways that you can reasonably avoid temptations and triggers when it comes to eliminating binge eating; however, you are going to need to focus just as much on your mindset as you do on your behaviors if you want to truly change. This is where meditation is going to help you really begin to start engaging in proper portion control so that you are no longer at risk of binge eating anymore. With meditation and hypnosis, you can begin to resolve the deep subconscious reasons behind your binge eating behaviors so that you have an easier time actually adhering to your changes. The more you engage in this deep healing, the easier it is going to be for you to make conscious and mindful changes in your eating habits, too.

As you use meditation and hypnosis to help you stop binge eating, you also need to focus on actually intentionally avoiding temptations and triggers. There are many practical ways that you can mindfully eliminate these temptations and triggers from your life. For example, you might intentionally stop buying the types of foods that you regularly binge eat so that the temptation no longer exists to begin with. You might also make sure that you eat on a consistent schedule so that you are no longer fasting to the point of being so hungry that you cannot stop yourself. If that is hard for you, picking up habits like meal prepping is a great opportunity for you to prevent yourself from waiting too long between meals and then binge eating as a way to make up for missing out on foods.

Another important way to start overcoming binge eating is to recognize that emotions can be a major trigger. In recognizing that, you can choose to identify and enlist new coping methods to help you navigate emotions in a healthier way that does not include binge eating. This way, you are more likely to manage your emotions with proper emotional management tools, rather than trying to numb yourself with the satisfaction that you get from snacking on junk foods.

If you find that anything else not listed here tends to be a temptation or trigger for you to binge eat, make sure that you remain aware of it and that you start offsetting it by changing your habits and behaviors. The more you can become aware of your own patterns and cycles, the easier it will be for you to find ways to overcome these patterns and cycles so that you can have a healthier relationship with food.

CHAPTER 16:

How Does Intermittent Fasting Work.

Although our ancestors were aware of the benefits of fasting, they did not have access to the scientific data we have today. In a culture where science is the standard for analysis of what is safe and effective, an intermittent fasting lifestyle would be shorthanded if it was lacking scientific verification of its validity. As fasting diets enter the mainstream, scientific communities are more inclined to research the practice, which, in turn, will allow the general public access to the information and results. A quick internet search will show a handful of studies, and there are surely more to come.

The physical results from an intermittent fasting routine are generally attributed to the calorie restriction that is at the heart of the practice. On the surface, this makes a lot of sense. Eat less food, lose more weight. This may suffice as an explanation for your everyday person, but studies have shown that a more complex equation is at work. Simply eating less and finding your desired results would be miraculous. It is obviously true that other factors that come into play, these factors include your mindset, genetics, stress, and exercise routine. One simple change is not going to completely transform your life. Along with the popular results of weight loss, intermittent fasting has been shown to combat many other unfavorable health risks. This list is quite expansive but let's touch on a few important ones.

Longevity

There have been studies showing that there is a link between fasting and longevity. This has been examined in lab-controlled settings as well as in the greater world. Many indigenous cultures that have a regular fasting routine built into their society have been shown to have some of the oldest living people on earth. Maintaining a healthy weight is the key to a long and successful life and intermittent fasting has been linked to weight loss through a sort of resetting of the circadian rhythms. These rhythms ensure that the body is balanced. When these rhythms are out of sync, diseases and sickness are more likely to manifest. Studies in mice have shown there is less of a risk for metabolic disease in subjects that had a restricted calorie diet, a phenomenon that translates to humans as well. Another incredible effect of fasting is the regulation of hormone secretion. Hormone regulation is linked to the circadian rhythms but in particular growth hormone secretion is positively affected by intermittent fasting, which in turn may be linked to IF's great influence on long life.

Digestive

It is a long list of beneficial health results that intermittent fasting boasts. The list above barely scratches the surface of the body's natural ability to heal itself with the help of intermittent fasting. Digestive relief is very prominent with newly adopted fasting routines. This is a result of giving your digestive system plenty of rest in between intake windows. Essentially, when we go to sleep, our digestive function stops and rests until we intake calories again. So, if one were to fast in the morning time, they would be giving their digestive functions some extra time to rest and repair itself. Setting a consistent intake window will allow us to build a relationship with our bodies. We become aware of our body's patterns, working with it to ensure regularity. This syncs up with the other bodily functions that we have effectively "reset", resulting in a full mind-body remake, a balance that we can then maintain throughout our lives.

The Brain

We have seen what physically takes place in the body while fasting but what about the more subtle effects? What about what happens in our brain? We should state here that we shouldn't confuse the brain and mind as one and the same. For our intentions in this book, the brain will be referred to as the physical effects that take place in our brain and the mind will refer to our perception and attitude. This being said, we need to look at the brain to fully understand the reactions that intermittent fasting induces. As mentioned above, hormone regulation is a huge benefit of fasting. This regulation takes place in the brain. As the control center of all of our bodily functions, the brain is at the forefront of our health concerns. With intermittent fasting showing such great influence on our brains, we once again find that the beneficial aspects cannot be ignored.

The brain is the epicenter of our entire physical existence wherein our physical and emotional state is dependent on. Seeing how fasting assists in some of the most important bodily functions, we need to reexamine what we have been taught about diet and food. Breaking away from societal standards that suggest an unbalanced and dangerous diet is imperative to achieve the results we desire. We can do this by focusing on our body's natural healing methods. Our body signals to our brain when it is in need. By fasting, we send a signal suggesting that we have no immediate intake of calories. This will trigger the brain to take action, reducing metabolic rates to conserve energy and fat reserves. With no immediate source of energy in the form of recently eaten foods, the body will burn fat reserves. This natural function, combined with a healthy diet and exercise, has shown to be a very safe way to lose weight.

The Heart

At one time in human history, the heart was thought to be the center of all emotional function. Science has proven otherwise, and we know now that the heart's most important function is regulation of our blood flow, distributing nutrients to the entire body. Heart disease has been a common source of illness and death. Unsurprisingly, the reasons for heart disease are combatted by an intermittent fasting routine. Unbalanced blood pressure, high cholesterol, diabetes, and obesity are the main causes of heart disease, and intermittent fasting has been shown to help regulate these symptoms. The "resetting" effect of fasting has assisted the functions of the heart repair and sync up with the rest of the body.

The Liver

Our liver is the filtration system of our body. If the liver is not functioning properly, then, we are left with toxins and other unwanted junk inside of us. The liver produces bile as well, a substance that assists with digestion in the intestines. If our livers are not in check, then many of the benefits of intermittent fasting can be jeopardized. Through the restriction of calories, we allow the liver ample time to do its job. With no toxins to filter, the liver can focus on its own healing capabilities. Also, during calorie restriction, one study found that the liver releases protein that regulates the liver's functions. The regulation and balancing of these natural functions are the keys to much of intermittent fasting's effectiveness.

Other Key Benefits

All the scientific evidence suggests just what many of our ancestors assumed, fasting is quite beneficial, if not mandatory, in the regulation of our body's natural healing functions. This is no small feat for any dietary practice, let alone a free and natural one. Along with the listed benefits above for our major organs, there are even more positive effects from including a fasting routine in our day to day lives. Here are some examples of IF's wonderful results:

- Assists with growth hormone secretion. Similar effects may be obtained through the consumption of supplements like HGH but the effectiveness of these supplements is debatable. Also, wouldn't a free and natural regulation of growth hormones be favored?

- Offers the body assistance with energy production by promoting the creation of mitochondria, the power sources inside of our cells. More energy will help maintain exercise routines and any other activities that require attentiveness and physical movement.

- Calorie restriction leaves the body no choice but to use fat reserves instead of seeking sugars from recent meals to burn. Fat cells are recognized as cleaner energy than carbohydrates and sugars. This will reduce the production of free radicals which have been linked to cancer through the oxidation of cells.

-       Reduces inflammation. Inflammation can damage cells and lead to immune diseases and similar other illness. Intermittent fasting can help care for damaged cells when ketones are produced through the burning of fat cells. Ketones help combat inflammation.

-       Fasting may also save the body from becoming intolerant to insulin. This may cause insulin to be produced excessively or not produce enough, resulting in diabetic symptoms.

These amazing benefits of IF cannot be ignored. The potential to naturally heal the body and restore organ health is unfounded by any other practice. But with these beneficial effects, many negative misconceptions arise. These misconceptions get propagated online and into the minds of thousands of people, thought to be true, but there is no scientific backing to validate the claims.

Common Misconceptions about Intermittent Fasting

Below are common misconceptions about intermittent fasting:

Fasting allows you to eat unhealthily

Many believe that if you fast sometimes, then you can eat whatever you want and remain healthful. This simply is not the case. Your body needs high-quality sources of nutrients. Sure, you receive some sustenance from a pizza, but these are rarely high-quality nutrients. To be healthy your body needs a variety of foods. Simply fasting then eating fast food in between fasts is not a healthy diet and can actually contradict the benefits of your intermittent fasting.

Fasting is the same as starving

This is a popular talking point for people who advocate against fasting of any type. While fasting can burn stored fat reserves, to be actually starving yourself you would need to use all of your stored sources of energy, and this is hardly even possible to do without getting ill, not to mention that fasting is intentionally restricting calories versus starving which is involuntary. Rest assured that you will not starve yourself if you take the needed measures to develop a safe and healthy intermittent fasting routine.

Fasting can destroy muscle

This is one of the more far-fetched myths in popular culture. When your body has not quick energy to burn, it turns to stored fat cells for fuel, not your muscles. While muscles can become weak and deteriorate in an unhealthy body, this is only in extreme cases where an individual is actually starved or have protein deficiencies. A balanced and mindful intermittent fasting routine is not going to negatively affect your muscles directly.

Fasting works for everyone

Many advocates of intermittent fasting sell it as the holy grail of health. But to realistic, fasting is not for everyone. As we have mentioned, not one lifestyle is going to work for everyone. Many people have illnesses or genetic predispositions that keep them from being able to fast, which is not uncommon throughout the world. Fasting may not work for you so do your research and consult a physician if you are unsure whether or not an intermittent fasting practice is right for you.

CHAPTER 17:

Chakra Guided Meditation

Your seven chakras are located along your spine and represent the seven energetic meridians that connect your body to your spiritual energy. Although they are rooted in spiritual energy and the unseen, your chakras have a huge impact on your physical wellbeing. This includes your ability to create and maintain a healthy body shape and physique. If you want to have your healthiest body in every way possible, you must incorporate spiritual energy work into your practice. This way, you can ensure that you are creating the energetic wellbeing that you need and that you deserve.

We are going to explore what your chakras are, how they affect weight loss, practical steps you can take to nurture your chakras, alternative strategies you can use to heal your chakras, and two important meditations you can use to help your chakras. Our goal here will be to create spiritual wellness within your emotions, mind, body, and soul so that you are able to let go of anything that may be preventing you from losing weight and keeping it off

What Are Your Chakras and How Do They Affect Weight Loss?

Your chakras are seven meridians located along your spine. They include your: root, sacral, solar plexus, heart, throat, third eye, and crown chakras. Each chakra represents a certain part of your mental, emotional, physical, and spiritual wellbeing. Ideally, when all of your chakras have been nurtured and balanced, you will find yourself experiencing complete health within your mind, emotions, body, and soul. This means that in addition to feeling grounded and balanced, you will also notice that your physical body actually begins to operate in optimal health. This includes anything and everything relating to your ability to lose weight and create and maintain a healthy and fit body that serves you.

Many cultures and healers, such as hypnosis masters, will tell you that if you focus on the wellbeing of each of your seven chakras, you will have a complete and structured guide for maintaining your wellness overall. They also insist that if you truly want to lose weight and have your healthiest body possible, educating yourself on and taking care of your chakras is crucial to your wellbeing. This is because your chakras are tangible points within your body, but they are also pointing that represent a bigger picture in your general wellbeing, and in all ways. For weight loss specifically, having healthy chakras means that you are not holding onto anything emotionally, mentally, physically, or spiritually that may be preventing you from having a healthier body. This means that you will release any traumas, negative thoughts, energies, and unhelpful habits or behaviors that may be negatively interrupting your physical wellbeing.

In order to better understand each of your chakras and how they contribute to weight loss and general wellbeing, let's take a brief look at each of your seven chakras.

Root Chakra: Your first chakra is your root chakra, located by the base of your tail bone and represented by the color red. This chakra reflects your physical stability, survival, and instincts. When it is imbalanced, you may retain weight as a way to "guarantee" your survival, sort of like a bear carrying weight to preserve his survival through the winter.

Sacral Chakra: Your second chakra is your sacral chakra, and it is located three finger-widths below your navel. This chakra is represented by the color orange. Carrying some extra weight around your sacral chakra is natural for women of childbearing years, however having too much weight can be unhealthy. Extra weight in this area is often linked to sexual health or sexual trauma.

It is represented by the color yellow. This chakra represents your feelings of personal power and personal strength. If you have repeatedly had your personal power taken from you or threatened, you may carry extra weight on your body as a way to protect yourself from those who have hurt you in the past. This is often seen as a "barrier" that protects you from the abuse of others. An imbalanced solar plexus chakra does not necessarily mean that you will carry more weight around your mid-section, as this weight may be distributed anywhere across your body.

Heart Chakra: Your fourth chakra is your heart chakra, it is located in the middle of your chest, and it is represented by the color green. Your heart chakra represents your feelings and your emotions. If you are carrying weight due to a lethargic heart chakra, this means that you are carrying emotional burdens that are "too heavy" for you and that need to be released so that you can let go of the extra weight of these burdens.

Throat Chakra: Your fifth chakra is your throat chakra, and it is located at the base of your throat, in that indented space where your throat meets your chest. Your throat chakra is represented by the color blue. Your throat chakra reflects your ability to communicate, including your ability to speak and your ability to hear what others have been saying to you. Your throat chakra may become imbalanced if you are regularly saying unkind things, or if you are regularly hearing unkind things, both of which can lead to you wanting to protect yourself with extra weight to "block" the pain.

Third Eye Chakra: Your third eye chakra is the sixth located between your eyebrows and up about 1-2 finger widths. This chakra is represented by the color indigo. Rarely will an imbalanced third eye chakra lead to weight gain, although an imbalanced third eye can indicate that you are experiencing imbalance elsewhere in your body. Symptoms of imbalance include nightmares, headaches, and struggling to see the entire truth of your life. One way this may translate to wellness could be in your inability to see your own beauty and the reality that you are more than just your body, particularly if you are struggling with body image issues and self-esteem.

Crown Chakra: Located at the crown of your head, directly over your spine, is your seventh chakra. The crown chakra is represented by the color violet. An imbalanced crown chakra means that you are not connected to the divine, which may lead to feelings of loneliness, isolation, or depression, all of which can encourage people to engage in unhealthy behaviors surrounding their wellness.

By balancing each of your seven chakras, you increase your likelihood of being able to effortlessly lose weight in a way that looks and feels good. Through this, you are not only going to create the body image that you want, but you are also going to be able to create the wellness that you desire so that you can genuinely feel happy and healthy in your life. This is imperative when losing weight, as many people do not realize that happiness is not inherently attached to weight loss, but instead to a willingness to accept yourself and respect and support yourself in all ways.

How Integrating Chakra Work Will Help You Lose Weight

Integrating chakra work can help you lose weight by essentially helping you let go of anything that may be preventing you from losing weight, while also fostering habits that help you maintain a healthy weight. Many people find that in choosing to work with their chakras, they discover a healthy and effective structure for how they can approach their wellness as a whole. In order to introduce you to this structure and give you some ideas for how you can integrate your chakras into your wellness and weight loss, let's explore each chakra individually and what you can do to create your desires through that chakra itself.

Your root chakra represents survival and instincts, which means that it connects with your primal subconscious in the deepest way possible. Learning to heal your fears around survival and wellbeing is a great way to allow your instincts to stop instinctively harboring extra weight on your body. This particular symptom often arises when people have grown up in poverty, or in a way that meant they struggled to have access to food or other necessities of survival. Creating a life where you can safely and consistently access healthy food and trusting that your food supply will not run out is a great way to start letting go of habits related to food hoarding and excess eating caused by a fear of survival.

Your sacral chakra represents your sexual urges and energy, as well as your cravings and desires. In order to integrate sacral chakra work into energy loss, you need to balance this chakra so that you can learn how to delay pleasure and desire. This way, you will be less likely to excessively indulge in cravings in order to meet your desires, and when you do choose to mindfully indulge, you will derive far more pleasure from your indulgence. Creating this balance will also help you release any fears you may have around "having enough" and "being enough" so that you can feel more at peace with yourself, your desires, and your desirability.

Your solar plexus chakra represents your personal power and confidence, which is something that many people who are unhappy with their body tend to struggle with. Learning to integrate your solar plexus chakra work by becoming more confident in yourself and more certain in your worthiness is a great way to release any weight or blocked energy that you may be carrying in your solar plexus chakra. As you create this balance, you will find yourself naturally building a body and a life that you feel more comfortable in and confident about.

Your heart chakra represents your emotions, which are something that many people struggle with. Becoming more attuned with your emotions and healing any emotional trauma or pain that you may be carrying is a good way for you to release anything that may be causing you to hold onto weight through your emotions. You will likely find that as you heal, your emotions, energy, and motivation come far more naturally and effortlessly for you.

Your throat chakra represents your ability to communicate and can have a negative impact on your weight when you have been repeatedly told unkind things about yourself, or you have said unkind things about yourself or others on a consistent basis. Learning to have healthier communication and to speak in a more positive and loving tone toward yourself and others is an important step in healing your mindset and laying the foundation for wellness in every way possible. Remember: your mind is the foundation of your entire reality and identity. Healing your communication abilities and habits will help you lay the foundation for healthier communication, a healthier identity, and a healthier reality. You can do this both by changing the way you speak about yourself and others and setting boundaries around how you are willing to allow others to speak about you.

CHAPTER 18:

Medical and Non-Medical Weight Loss Treatments.

A s the problem of weight problems continues to grow, a substantial number of people are taking extreme action to fight this condition. Many obese victims are also reverting to surgical treatment as a fast solution, although a variety of other weight reduction treatments are offered today.

Obesity Statistics

With current researches and equivalent outcomes, providing a grim picture, obesity statistics have developed right into a bright and existing risk. This common issue is observed to have substantially risen no matter the fellow age, gender, financial standing, or race.

In the past years alone, nations that were once hailed for health policies such as the United States, Canada, and England have revealed troubling numbers on climbing obesity. Weight problems is a health and wellness condition noted with an extraordinarily high percentage of body fat. Obesity and weight problems statistics have placed the lives of millions in jeopardy and have the potential to continue to produce new patients experiencing diabetes mellitus, high blood pressure, osteoarthritis, and sleep apnea.

Tracking obesity is primarily based on the Body Mass Index (BMI), where a recognized cutoff factor acts as the guide to identify whether one is overweight or overweight. Weight problems data show numerous factors associated with the disease, such as grown-up weight problems, childhood years excessive weight, consuming routines, the occurrence of hypertension, high blood cholesterol, gallbladder, and cardiovascular disease, and cancer. The rate of adjustment of obesity occurrence for many years has increased.

Obesity stats also show a rise in mortality price connected with excessive weight as obese individuals have a 50-100% increased threat of fatality from all reasons. Even those moderately overweight people have their life span shortened by 2 to 5 years. Weight problems stats also show that it is a lot more common as one age. Over 28% of males and 27% of females aged 16-24 are overweight in the world, along with regarding 76% of men and 68% of ladies in between 55 and 64. Worldwide, weight problems are a primary threat lurking in most homes today.

Non-Medical Treatments

Therapy for weight problems will undoubtedly be most successful if you develop a long-term strategy with your physician. A sensible goal could be to start making way of living changes by boosting physical activity and limiting calories. It is expected that a specific with a BMI fantastic than or equivalent to 30, in addition to those with a BMI of 25.0-29.9 in enhancement to 2 or more illness risk factors have to attempt to slim down either with clinical or non-medical treatments. Non-medical ways are:

By sticking to a program of workout, diet plan, and behavior therapy, one complies with a specific regimen for a discrete-time period, applying behavioral and nutritional changes that can be sustained indefinitely to advertise health and wellness.

Exercise-The most significant advantage of physical activity is its facilitative activity in weight loss upkeep.

Behavior change - This kind of therapy offers clients a collection of concepts and methods to facilitate their adherence to the diet and activity objectives that they have set on their own.

Over-the-counter organic weight reduction supplements - These supplements are normally referred to as 'fat burners' and work by boosting the body's metabolic process. Physicians have commonly prescribed these weight-loss supplements, though the progression has always been very closely monitored. These supplements are actively prevented due to a lack of labeling of ingredients on these items, and they have the capacity to create a drastic boost in blood stress and heart issues.

Medical Intervention includes:

Medicinal Interventions - As BMI or disease risk boosts, even more, extensive choices are offered for the therapy of obesity. 2 medications - sibutramine (Reductil) and orlistat (Xenical) - are authorized drugs for the induction and upkeep of secure weight-loss.

Sibutramine - is a mixed serotonin-norepinephrine reuptake prevention that is related to records of boosted satiation (i.e., volume).

Orlistat -. Individuals are negatively enhanced to eat a low-fat diet plan since refraining from doing so can generate unfavorable stomach occasions that consist of oily feces, flatus with discharge, and fecal necessity.

Surgical Interventions - Bariatric surgery, the most intensive therapy for weight problems, is suitable just for those people with a BMI e35-40 in the presence of comorbidities. Typically, people that seek bariatric surgical treatment need to have exhausted the extra conservative weight management choices without acceptable outcomes. The two most usual procedures entail isolating a small pouch of the stomach with a line of staples, thus dramatically limiting food intake. The operations are:

- Vertical banded gastroplasty

- Stomach bypass

Acupuncture - While acupuncture for weight-loss has been around for ages currently, it has just recently been used for treating individuals for weight reduction or excessive weight. It functions by curbing the client's hunger, inhibits yearnings for food, removes excess water in the body, and stimulates the pituitary gland to burn off added calories. It takes advantage of acupuncture ear staples for fat burning. The process is not a medically confirmed, and while it might function for some, there are no guaranteed results.

Hypnosis - Hypnotic sessions enable one to break devoid of pre-formed principles, and self recognizes oneself. This mode discovers the various reasons the body is lugging around those additional pounds and works in the direction of launching extra emotional luggage. It can assist us in escaping from negative thoughts, boost metabolic rate, release negative obese habits in addition to lower sugar cravings and food addictions.

Liposuction surgery - Is a surgery that eliminates excess fat or localized fat down payments with a suction process. It can also modify physique.

166

CHAPTER 19:

Getting Started with Iron Yoga

With Iron Yoga principles under your belt, you're nearly ready to get started. Think about your goals as you begin to train for your Iron Yoga session. What do you hope to do by doing your Iron Yoga? Need to lose any weight? After a long day at the workplace, you want to find a way to decompress? Want to get stronger and leaner? Need to only become more physically fit? Write down your priorities after you're clear about your plans for action. It will help you find the time to practice Iron Yoga for years to come, and keep you inspired.

When to practice

No right time to do Iron Yoga when To Do. You need to find a time that works particularly for you. Whatever time you want to exercise, make sure that you give your body enough time to digest food—90 minutes after a snack, or 2 hours after a heavier meal. If you do the first thing in the morning, you should have an empty stomach that will not interfere with your workout.

They will preferably practice Iron Yoga two or three times a week. The initial goal will help you familiarize yourself with the special Iron Yoga sequences. When you're new to yoga then it's going to take some time to master the poses. Unless you have been doing certain forms of yoga, then you can typically catch up a little quicker with the technique.

What You Need (Equipment)

One of Iron Yoga's best aspects is that you don't need tons of costly workout facilities, gizmos or gadgets. You will find just about anything in your local sporting goods store listed here. What's more, you don't need a lot of space to practice Iron Yoga — it can fit well in a classroom, tiny studio apartment or basement.

Yoga mat: A mat helps prevent the body from falling onto the surface. Also, if you're doing carpeting work, I recommend you buy a pad. Many carpeting can be as slick as a smooth pavement.

Dumbbells: Iron Yoga is not about the heavy weight lifting. I recommend a pair of dumbbells, each weighing 2 or 3 pounds, when you start out first. You should increase the weight to 4 or 5 pounds after you feel confident with the movements. The emphasis is not on the sum of dumbbell weight but the strength of the link between your mind and muscle.

Mirror: I advise to practice in front of a mirror for those new to yoga. Alignment and posture in yoga are extremely necessary. It will give you an opportunity to see if your body is in the right place. Finding yourself in a mirror will also help you with balancing poses and weight lifting exercises in the right manner.

Clothing: You should wear light, comfortable and breathable clothing so that your body can feel unrestricted as you walk.

Bare feet: As with all types of yoga, you can perform Iron Yoga with bare feet. You need to be able to hold steady without sliding to get the correct traction in the standing and balancing poses. Wearing socks lets you slip around.

A quiet space: Select a room or area that is quiet and free from interruptions as much as possible. A noisy television or ringing phone will distract you from the attention you'll need for the session.

Practicing Safely

Iron Yoga's most basic rule — and every form of yoga in that respect — is listening to your body. Never take a pose to a point that risks your body getting hurt. The depth of a pose is regulated by proper yogic breathing, and should only go to a point the body can tolerate. A pose should never make any part of the body feel pain and discomfort. The Iron Yoga workout emphasizes perfect posture and alignment, correct form execution with each weight-training exercise, and guided movement flows from one pose to another. Learn to recognize the difference between muscle burning caused by deepening a pose or intensifying peak contraction and knee, leg, feet, thighs, back, shoulders, or elbow pain caused by executing a pose or weight-training exercise incorrectly. Muscle burning is good — and it is this sensation that will result in positive results in shaping, toning, and body sculpture. Joint pain is unpleasant during every workout, and must be stopped and prevented.

Modifications: Changes Any pose in Iron Yoga can be modified depending on your level of practical experience and your own physical limitations. I've mentioned some modifications for different

170

movements in the instructions. What you'll see later. In short, when you're doing a weight-training exercise, the best change is to simply put the dumbbells on the floor and perform the movement without weight.

When you have a particular condition that can affect your practice, take careful notice of the changes for the circumstances that follow.

Back pain: Back pain is usually caused by poor posture. Many of us work on computer typing for long periods of the day, or looking at computer screens. Heavy abdominals in conjunction with tight hamstrings can be a source, too. Believe it or not, stress is also a significant cause of back and neck pain. Iron Yoga's meditative and calming aspect will greatly help you relieve stress, particularly in those problematic areas.

The practice of Iron Yoga will aid by strengthening the muscles in the abs and lower back. The floor poses like Bow and Cow / Cat, are perfect to stretch your lower neck and back. Hamstring stretches like Standing will allow the lower back to be strengthened.

Modifications: during forward folding and stretching movements, you should be sure to bend your knees. Remember to execute each pose gently and stop immediately if you feel any strain to your lower back or neck.

Pregnancy: You must practice intense caution about practicing Iron Yoga during pregnancy. As you would during pregnancy, consult your doctor about every fitness program. If you have never practiced Iron Yoga, I recommend you wait before you start giving birth. If you've been doing Iron Yoga before your pregnancy, then I recommend that you quit during your first trimester—and make sure you limit the strength and length of the practice when you return in your second and third trimesters. Many of Iron Yoga's advantages to you and your baby are that it relaxes your whole body and relieves back problems.

Modifications: Deep forward bends, spinal twists and any position that puts pressure on your uterus should be avoided You will simply stop lying completely on your stomach. You should walk slowly and gently and avoid any leaps or rapid movements, as during pregnancy the joints will gradually become looser due to increased levels of certain hormones. Be careful not to exaggerate the muscles, because this may result in serious injury.

Seniors: Iron Yoga can be of great help to older people. One of Iron Yoga's most significant advantages is deep abdominal breathing, and concentration on breathing. Deep abdominal respiration opens the lungs and strengthens the respiratory system. In Iron Yoga, the strength exercises with light weights can help maintain strong bones and prevent bone loss (osteoporosis), particularly for women. Bone loss for women will actually start much earlier — in your thirties — so starting Iron Yoga really never gets too early. Good balance and stability are particularly important for seniors in helping prevent falls. The balancing poses like Tree and Eagle in are ideal for such skills growth.

Modifications: You can use a chair for the balancing poses, or stand for extra support against the wall.

Aligning with Your Body

One of the most important aspects of the Iron Yoga practice is to link your mind with a particular muscle and not just your breath. As I explain how each of the movements should be done, I ask you to "engage" a particular muscle or muscle group. In other words, you should develop a mental link to the muscle before you start working on it. This technique is very strong and has been used by many bodybuilders.

It's crucial that you understand some basic anatomy to help link your mind to your muscles. Some of you already know these basic body parts, but even so, take the time here to learn the names and positions of the muscles.

Know Your Body

One of the most important aspects of Iron Yoga practice is to link your mind to a particular muscle and not just your breath. As I explain how each of the movements should be done, I ask you to "engage" a particular muscle or muscle group. In other words, you should develop a mental link to the muscle before you start working on it. This technique is very strong and has been used by many bodybuilders.

It's crucial that you understand some basic anatomy to help link your mind to your muscles. Most of you already know these basic body parts, but even so, take the time here to learn the names and positions of the muscles.

Abs, Right and Left Obliques (Rectus Abdominis, Transverse Abdominis, Internal Obliques, External Obliques) This is a group of muscles forming the central area. Such muscles help to fine-tune your waist and to balance and secure your spine. The obliques aid motions such as spinning and side bending as well as gravity motions such as sitting up, running, and climbing. Boat, Half Moon, Oblique Crunch and Oblique Twist are aimed directly at the heart.

LATS (LatissimusDorsi)

The lats are the back's most extensive muscles. They stretch all the way from your pelvis by wrapping around the ribs to your shoulder blades. The weight-training exercises LatPulldown, Lat Pullback, and Row really help to develop these muscles.

TRAPS (Trapezius)

Traps are huge, triangular muscles, stretching from the base of your skull to about two-thirds of the way down the back. These muscles help you raise your arms, stretch your head and balance it. Often, they keep the shoulders squared. Weight-training exercises for the Shoulder Shrug and Upright Row target this area.

PECS (Pectoralis)

This group of muscles is found in the forehead and under the breasts. Once your hands are pressed together in front of your chest it flexes and rotates your muscles. Strengthening those muscles is important to help you stabilize your shoulders. You should consider the weight-training exercises Chest Press and Chest Flye especially helpful to toning and shaping your pecs. The poses in the Salutation to the Light, Plank and Chaturanga are also perfect for chest practice.

DELTS (Deltoids)

The delts form your shoulders and are composed of three muscles: anterior or front, medial or middle, and posterior or back. The delts help you spin your arms inside and out. The delts even help lift your arms to your body's forehead, hands, and rear. Strengthen your delts with the following exercises: Front Raise, Lateral Raise, Rear Lateral Raise, Reverse Flye, Shoulder Overhead Press and Modified Lateral Raise.

ROTATOR CUFFS

This is a group of muscles which are close to your shoulder area. The rotator cuff helps your shoulder joint to stabilise and rotate. The movements of the external / internal rotation help to target and reinforce this group of muscles.

CHAPTER 20:

Intuitive Eating Struggles

A dieter may say that a diet is a solution to all your problems, but an intuitive eater will tell you that all the answers you seek are within yourself. It is true, all the answers we seek are within us because it was designed by Mother Nature that way.

Call it a Buddha approach, but this is exactly what intuitive eating teaches us. The idea behind intuitive eating is to reconnect with our inner self, tune into it to let us guide ourselves with its wisdom and help us figure out a way to eat the right way.

Unlike traditional diets, intuitive eating allows its followers some wiggle room to interpret their body needs and execute them. This is what makes it such an ideal approach to eating. There are no limitations or bindings. However, it is the same flexibility that makes it so easy to give up on intuitive eating as most people consider it a failure as it doesn't make them lose weight. But it was never the actual goal of eating intuitively. Many people see it as unrealistic because there aren't any restrictions, which they consider a requisite to any diet form.

7 Mistakes You Are Making with Intuitive Eating

Did you know, the number one reason that all these misconceptions and myths form is because we make multiple mistakes with intuitive eating? As long as we don't understand the core concept, we will fail to practice and incorporate it into our daily lives and become an intuitive eater like we were when we were kids. Therefore, to put the above myths to rest, it is pivotal that we take a look at all the mistakes we make while trying to eat intuitively to be able to practice it better.

Mistake #1: Thinking You Can Eat Whatever You Want Whenever You Want

Yes, intuitive eating allows you to pick whichever food your body craves and wishes to eat, but it also reminds us to treat our body with honor and respect. How do you do that? By ensuring that you feed it with good nutrition. Now, if you are following the diet to the tee, you will stop craving junk food as you realize that it leaves you feeling lethargic and sluggish. You want to feel energetic, satisfied, and fulfilled which can only come from healthy eating and limiting the greasy, fatty, and "fast" food along the way.

Mistake #2: Not Giving Up the Diet Mentality

How many times will we have to remind you that intuitive eating isn't a diet? One of the primary reasons people give up on intuitive eating is because they see it as a means to lose weight. Yes, it helps in doing so but it was never its core intention. The core intention was to get in touch with our inner selves and let it take control of our eating choices and habits. If you didn't come with this intention in mind, then perhaps, it is true that it won't work for you.

You need to give up on the diet mentality, which also happens to be the first principle of intuitive eating. The more you cling to it, the lesser your chances of becoming an intuitive eater. You need to trust your body and let it guide you. You need to appreciate the way it looks rather than trying to change it with poor dietary choices that lead to health conditions and hormonal imbalances.

Yes, it may seem difficult to not think about the diet mentality or let it go, but you must if you wish to become an intuitive eater.

Mistake #3: Believing You Can't Lose Weight with Intuitive Eating

If you recently just came off a diet, your biggest worry right now must be if you will continue to lose weight or worse, will you regain all your lost weight. Here's the thing with intuitive eating, if you pay attention to your body's needs and only eat when you're moderately hungry and stop when you're moderately full, you will see the pointer on your weighing scale fall back. Moreover, since there will be no restrictions as to what you can eat, there will rarely be any cravings. If you continue down this road, you will also begin to notice that your body will stop craving for fun foods as it was naturally designed to function on fruits, veggies, nuts, and other nutritious foods.

All these aspects of intuitive eating make for a classic weight-loss recipe, doesn't it? So how can you not lose weight with it?

Mistake #4: Continuing with Food Restrictions

When eating intelligently, there are no restrictions on what you are eating and in what quantity as long as you eat when you're hungry and stop when you're full. There are no rules with intuitive eating which means you can quiet the food police that tell you what to eat and what not to eat. Try to eat more of the foods that pass the health test and are loaded with nutrients like vitamin, iron, Omega-3, and good carbs.

Besides, when you stop denying your body certain foods, it will also put an end to your cravings which often result in binge or emotional eating.

Mistake #5: You Disregard Physical Activity

Just because you are no longer keeping a check of calories with every meal doesn't give you the right to become a couch potato and give up exercising. Staying active is a crucial part of intuitive eating? You need to burn what you are eating and that means sweating up or making your heart race faster for at least 30 minutes per day. It doesn't have to be a hardcore, rigorous fitness regime, but definitely something that gets your blood gushing through your veins faster.

Start with something you enjoy doing, say walking and then pace it up to brisk walking and full-on jogging to build your stamina and improve your digestion and metabolic rate.

Mistake #6: Thinking it's About Failing or Succeeding

There is no concept of failure or success in intuitive eating. It isn't a race but rather a process that takes time and practice to learn and live by. Despite this, most people just assume that since they aren't losing weight, the diet is a failure and move onto another one. If you keep thinking this way about intuitive eating and stay focused on just the results, you will always be judging and critiquing your choices.

Intuitive eating isn't about perfectionism but rather continuing to progress towards a healthier lifestyle. So, don't be too critical of yourself and don't stand on the weighing scale every single day hoping for a miracle. The miracle is learning to listen to your internal messages.

Mistake #7: You Think You Have a Free Hand with Portions

Portion control may not be the core concept of intuitive eating, but there is a strong emphasis on stopping when you're full which almost the same thing is. Since intuitive eating isn't a "diet," many people believe there aren't any restrictions when it comes to portions. True, you can eat whatever you want but in a considerate amount. Though, don't go measuring how many bites you have taken. Listen to the inner cues that tell you when to stop. With time, you will notice how good you become at controlling your portions and stopping when you are no longer hungry.

Take Away

We looked at the many mistakes intuitive eaters make when they're just starting out. This consists of things like not knowing when to stop, thinking it is only about eating, not honoring your body with the right nutrition, and underestimating the importance of exercise.

CHAPTER 21:

Blasting Calories

We have all heard the word "calorie" and its relation to our body weight. Calories are contained in the foods we consume and are often misunderstood about how they affect us. In this topic, we seek to explain what they are, how to count them, and the best methods of blasting them to avoid weight gain.

What are Calories, and How Do They Affect Your Weight?

A calorie is a key estimating unit. For example, we use meters when communicating separation;' Usain Bolt went 100 meters in simply 9.5 seconds.' There are two units in this expression. One is a meter (a range unit), and the other is "second" (a period unit). Essentially, calories are additional units of physical amount estimation.

Many assume that a calorie is the weight measure (since it is oftentimes connected with an individual's weight). That is not precise, however. A calorie is a vitality unit (estimation). 1 calorie is proportional to the vitality expected to build the temperature by 1 degree Celsius to 1 kilogram of water.

Two particular sorts of calories come in: small calories and huge calories. Huge calories are the word connected to sustenance items.

You've likely observed much stuff on parcels (chocolates, potato chips, and so forth.) with' calorie scores.' Imagine the calorie score an incentive for a thing being' 100 cal.' this infers when you eat it, you will pick up about as much vitality (even though the calorie worth expressed and the amount you advantage from it is never the equivalent).

All that we eat has a particular calorie tally; it is the proportion of the vitality we eat in the substance bonds. B

These are mostly things we eat: starches, proteins, and fats. How about we take a gander at what number of calories 1 gram comprises of these medications: 1. Sugars 4 calories 2. Protein-3 calories. Fat–nine calories

Are my calories awful?

That is fundamentally equivalent to mentioning, "Is vitality awful for me?" Every single activity the body completes needs vitality. Everything takes vitality to stand, walk, run, sit, and even eat. In case you're doing any of these tasks, it suggests you're utilizing vitality, which mostly infers you're' consuming' calories, explicitly the calories that entered your body when you were eating some nourishment.

To sum things up, for you, NO... calories are not terrible.

Equalization is the way to finding harmony between what number of calories you devour and what number of calories you consume or use. On the off chance that you eat fewer calories and spend more, you will become dainty, while on the opposite side, on the off chance that you gobble up heaps of calories, however, you are a habitually lazy person, you will in the long run become stout at last.

Each movement we do throughout a day will bring about certain calories being spent. Here is a little rundown of the absolute most much of the time performed exercises, just as the number of calories consumed while doing them.

Step by Step Instructions to Count Calories

You have to expend fewer calories than you consume to get thinner.

This clamor is simple in principle. Be that as it may, it very well may be hard to deal with your nourishment admission in the contemporary sustenance setting. Calorie checking is one approach to address this issue and is much of the time used to get more fit. Hearing that calories don't make a difference is very common, and tallying calories is an exercise in futility. Nonetheless, calories tally with regards to your weight; this is a reality that, in science, analyses called overloading studies has been demonstrated on numerous occasions.

These examinations request that people deliberately indulge and after that, survey the impact on their weight and wellbeing. All overloading investigations have found that people are putting on weight when they devour a bigger number of calories than they consume.

This simple reality infers that calorie checking and limiting your utilization can be proficient in averting weight put on or weight reduction as long as you can stick to it. One examination found that health improvement plans, including calorie including brought about a normal weight reduction of around 7 lbs. (3.3 kg) more than those that didn't.

Primary concern: You put on weight by eating a larger number of calories than you consume. Calorie tallying can help you expend fewer calories and get more fit.

How Many Calories Do You Have to Eat?

What number of calories you need depends on factors, for example, sex, age, weight, and measure of activity? For example, a 25-year-old male competitor will require a bigger number of calories than a non-practicing 70-year-elderly person. In case you're endeavoring to get in shape, by eating not exactly your body consumes off, you'll have to construct a calorie deficiency. Utilize this adding machine to decide what number of calories you ought to expend every day (opening in crisp tab). This number cruncher depends on the condition of Mifflin-St Jeor, an exact method to evaluate calorie prerequisites.

How to Reduce your Caloric Intake for Weight Loss

Bit sizes have risen, and a solitary dinner may give twofold or triple what the normal individual needs in a sitting at certain cafés. "Segment mutilation" is the term used to depict enormous parts of sustenance as the standard. It might bring about weight put on and weight reduction. In general, people don't evaluate the amount they spend. Tallying calories can help you battle indulging by giving you a more grounded information of the amount you expend.

In any case, you have to record portions of sustenance appropriately for it to work. Here are a couple of well-known strategies for estimating segment sizes: Scales: Weighing your sustenance is the most exact approach to decide the amount you eat. This might be tedious, in any case, and isn't constantly down to earth.

Estimating cups: Standard estimations of amount are, to some degree, quicker and less complex to use than a scale, yet can some of the time be tedious and unbalanced.

Examinations: It's quick and easy to utilize correlations with well-known items, especially in case you're away from home. It's considerably less exact, however.

Contrasted with family unit items, here are some mainstream serving sizes that can help you gauge your serving sizes: 1 serving of rice or pasta (1/2 a cup): a PC mouse or adjusted bunch.

- 1 Meat serving (3 oz): a card deck.

- 1 Fish serving (3 oz): visit book.

- 1 Cheese serving (1.5 oz): a lipstick or thumb size.

- 1 Fresh organic product serving (1/2 cup): a tennis ball.

- 1 Green verdant vegetable serving (1 cup): baseball.

- 1 Vegetable serving (1/2 cup): a mouse PC.

- 1 Olive oil teaspoon: 1 fingertip.

- 2 Peanut margarine tablespoons: a ping pong ball.

Calorie tallying, notwithstanding when gauging and estimating partitions, isn't a careful science.

In any case, your estimations shouldn't be thoroughly spot-on. Simply guarantee that your utilization is recorded as effectively as would be prudent. You ought to be mindful to record high-fat as well as sugar things, for example, pizza, dessert, and oils. Under-recording these meals can make an enormous qualification between your genuine and recorded utilization. You can endeavor to utilize scales toward the begin to give you a superior idea of what a segment resembles to upgrade your evaluations. This should help you to be increasingly exact, even after you quit utilizing them.

More Tips to Assist in Caloric Control

Here are 5 more calorie tallying tips:

• Get prepared: get a calorie tallying application or web device before you start, choose how to evaluate or gauge parcels, and make a feast plan.

• Read nourishment marks: Food names contain numerous accommodating calorie tallying information. Check the recommended segment size on the bundle.

• Remove the allurement: dispose of your home's low-quality nourishment. This will help you select more advantageous bites and make hitting your objectives easier.

• Aim for moderate, steady loss of weight: don't cut too little calories. Even though you will get in shape all the more rapidly, you may feel terrible and be less inclined to adhere to your arrangement.

• Fuel your activity: Diet and exercise are the best health improvement plans. Ensure you devour enough to rehearse your vitality.

Effective Methods for Blasting Calories

To impact calories requires participating in exercises that urge the body to utilize vitality. Aside from checking the calories and guaranteeing you eat the required sum, consuming them is similarly basic for weight reduction. Here, we examine a couple of techniques that can enable you to impact our calories all the more viably.:

1. Indoor cycling: mccall states that around 952 calories for each hour ought to be at 200 watts or higher. On the off chance that the stationary bicycle doesn't demonstrate

watts: "this infers you're doing it when your indoor cycling instructor educates you to switch the opposition up!" he proposes.

2. Skiing: around 850 calories for every hour depends on your skiing knowledge. Slow, light exertion won't consume nearly the same number of calories as a lively, fiery exertion is going to consume. To challenge yourself and to consume vitality? Attempt to ski tough.

3. Rowing: approximately 816 calories for every hour. The benchmark here is 200 watts; mccall claims it ought to be at a "fiery endeavor." many paddling machines list the showcase watts. Reward: rowing is additionally a stunning back exercise.

4. Jumping rope: about 802 calories for each hour this ought to be at a moderate pace— around 100 skips for each moment—says mccall. Attempt to begin with this bounce rope interim exercise.

5. Kickboxing: approximately 700 calories for every hour. Also, in this class are different sorts of hand to hand fighting, for example,

muay thai. With regards to standard boxing, when you are genuine in the ring (a.k.a. Battling another individual), the biggest calorie consumption develops. Be that as it may, many boxing courses additionally incorporate cardio activities, for example, hikers and burpees, so your pulse will in the long run increment more than you would anticipate. What's more, hello, before you can get into the ring, you need to start someplace, isn't that so?

6. Swimming: approximately 680 calories for each hour freestyle works, however as mccall says, you should go for a vivacious 75 yards for each moment. For an easygoing swimmer, this is somewhat forceful. (butterfly stroke is significantly progressively productive if you extravagant it.)

7. Outdoor bicycling: approximately 680 calories for each hour biking at a fast, lively pace will raise your pulse, regardless of whether you are outside or inside. Add to some rocky landscape and mountains and gets significantly more calorie consuming.

The volume of calories devoured is straightforwardly proportionate to the measure of sustenance, just like the kind of nourishment an individual expends. The best way to lessen calories is by being cautious about what you devour and captivating in dynamic physical exercises to consume overabundance calories in your body.

CHAPTER 22:

The Steps of Grain Detox

The Wheat Belly Grain Detox starts with the idea that the foods we are told (again and again) will dominate our diet — grains — need to be eliminated in all their varied forms altogether. This is the first major step to regaining control of weight and health. This means eliminating the appetite-stimulating effects of cookies and bagels, autoimmune disease–triggering effects of multigrain bread, animal crackers' behavior-distortion and learning impairment, and breakfast cereal gastrointestinal disruption. It might sound dramatic; some might even say it is unlikely. Others say it can lead to food shortages, trouble managing social environments, being thrown out of the country club, friends not talking to you anymore, having to confess to your priest, even malnutrition and disability. None of this really is valid.

When you're aware of a few simple rules in your newly empowered grain-free existence, I expect you'll find this lifestyle totally manageable, empowering, delicious and safe. Yeah, efforts can take some to get used to, such as as asking restaurant waiting staff about the ingredients in the dishes you order, but these efforts are minimal and easy to accomplish. And that's what you need to do to get exceptional power over appetite and health.

To make the transition to grain-free living a digestible process for you, even though your life is hectic and full of other commitments, I have broken it down into three parts that are bite-sized, grain-free, sugar-free. With this lifestyle the three steps to get started are:

1. Dispose of all grains.

2. Eat organic foods which are single-ingredient.

3. Manage Carbohydrates.

That is so plain. Sure, there are more steps to be taken to restore body-wide fitness. So, it's just that easy to switch from an inexperienced, weak, inflamed, weight-accumulating, disease-causing, grain-filled diet to a health-enhancing, performance-enhancing, feel-great-again, grain-free diet.

When we go back to eating foods that we are adapted to consume (since grains were added just a moment ago, anthropologically speaking), there are no concerns about saturated fat or fiber, there is nothing to be suggested, no one needs to count calories, and there are certainly no products made from grains. We leave questions about portion size or overeating behind. We return to foods that allowed humans to live and prosper on Earth for more than 99% of our time, when overweight and society diseases (such as diabetes, hypertension, and autoimmune diseases) were unknown, until we wrongly turned to desperate grains as a source of calories when nothing else was available; grains were then used as food for food, gr.

Re-creating such a new, but genuinely ancient, pre-grain diet means making provisions for the modern options that we are faced with, as we are not going to spear wild boar or dig in the dirt for wild roots. Therefore, in locations like supermarkets we need to know how to handle their nearest modern counterparts.

We start with the first move which is essential, inevitable and utterly necessary.

STEP 1: Dispose of All Grains

We begin by eliminating the unexpected and shocking cause of so many problems: no, not your nit-picky mother-in-law or the unhealthy sports television viewing habits of your spouse, but grains. It is not unusual for humans to get over half of their daily calories from grains. Eliminating them is a major challenge to shopping, dining and cooking habits. But I don't know of anything — extreme exercise, prescription drugs, nutritional supplements, enemas washing, meditation, a year in a monastery — that can equal the benefits of eliminating these health disrupters.

Grain removal is by far the most critical step in detoxification, and of course the next few steps must follow this crucial first step. By banishing grains, you remove the appetite-stimulating effects of grain-derived opiates, which encourage junk carbohydrate consumption. You will also remove gastrointestinal toxins that change the sense of taste in grains. Without these effects, your hunger will diminish, you'll spend much less time starving (if you're hungry at all), and your sense of taste will be resurrected. You will no longer find fine, even sickeningly sweet, former goodies and you will enjoy more nutritious foods. For starters, you'll discover that Brussels sprouts and blueberries have flavor dimensions you've never encountered before. The physiological changes you undergo in Step 1 promote the detoxification of the two subsequent phases.

Let me be very explicit about this: Exclude all grains. I am not referring to cut back. Save Friday I do not say every day. Though going back to grain-consuming ways in restaurants or friends' homes, I don't mean just at home. Just a little compromise will obstruct the progress entirely, interrupt the detoxification cycle, maintain the addictive and appetite-stimulating effects of the opiate and continue to promote inflammation. So, when I say "eliminate all grains," I mean 100 per cent without compromise, regardless of where you are, what other people think, or what day of the week it is. Before this crucial first step and going the full distance with it, you cannot excel in this lifestyle, because none of the other steps will follow or achieve the results you want. And let's think about how you can achieve this very critical first step and banish all of your life's grains.

Start with a Grain-Free Kitchen

I recommend that you start this lifestyle by developing a grain-free kitchen: set up a grain-free zone that includes your refrigerator, pantry and cabinet shelves cleaned from all grain foods. Store stores, fast food joints, and schools can be packed with them from top to bottom, but your personal kitchen is going to be a grain-free safe zone, a sanctuary for nutritious food.

Start by eliminating all obvious wheat flour sources such as bread, rolls, doughnuts, pasta, cookies, cake, pretzels, crackers, pancake mix, cereals for breakfast, crumbs and bagels. To save a few bucks on delivery of pizza or bakery goods, throw out all the coupons you have set aside. Then exclude from the ingredients all imported bottled, canned, packaged and frozen foods with wheat.

Next, tackle food containing barley. It includes all foods mentioned on the label with malt, as well as barley itself. (Beer and some other alcoholic drinks have grain problems) All rye foods, such as rye breads and rye crackers, will go as well. Now exclude all obvious sources of maize such as cob corn, canned corn, maize chips, tacos, and grits, as well as refined packaged foods made with obvious and not-so-obvious maize ingredients such as hydrolyzed maize starch and polenta.

Other grains, including oats, rice, millet, sorghum, amaranth, and tiff, are typically identified by their real names; remove these foods from the kitchen.

Conclusion

You look in the mirror and you are dissatisfied. Do you wish that your shape, your nose, your legs, your hair were like somebody else's? Why do we always compare ourselves? Why aren't we reconciled with our appearance? We have heard ad nauseam that we should love ourselves, despite our mistakes or flaws. This includes things related to our personality as well as our bodies. However, there are very few people who can accept and be content with themselves. It is not about not wanting to change. It is a commendable endeavor when one wants to achieve or retain their looks or care about looking more attractive.

At the same time, most people are much more critical, stricter with themselves than justified. They are continuously dissatisfied with themselves and don't see in the mirror what others see. Some girls feel a significant discomfort looking at each other, both because they don't like looking at each other in general, and because they don't like what they see. Where do these reactions come from?

What usually happens is that you don't look at yourself; you only see yourself with respect to that ideal of beauty that you have in your head. This is where dissatisfaction creeps in. It has to do with the theory of social confrontation. We compare ourselves with those we consider better than ourselves; self-esteem is negatively affected. We all have a model in the head, a term of comparison that we have built by looking at years of magazines, advertising, and movies with perfect Hollywood princesses. The mantra must become one and only one: there is no need for me to compare myself to that model because everybody is a unique, generous specimen, rich in the indications of what I am.

Life would be much simpler and happier if we could accept ourselves as we are. A lot of negative emotions would be released, we would have less stress, and more of the things that really matter come into view. The bottom line is, if we really need to change something, we can't do it until we make peace with the current state. This is a vicious circle.

The mind works, in effect, in a strange way. If we resist something, we get more of it.

After all, if we focus our attention on what is bad, we reinforce the bad. And what we pay the most attention to as we think about something will come true.

Everything that comes from you that relates to you is just yours: your feelings, your voice, your actions, your ears, your thighs, your hopes and fears. That's why you are unique. Be happy that you are different from anyone, that you look the way you do and that it is just you. Start to feel that it's your own body, not something separate that you need to live with.

Do you want your house to be just like anyone else's? Or do you love the little things that carry memories? Don't you love the atmosphere of your messy place after playing with your kids? And the plain curtain that you know you should replace, but which your mom sewed and looks so good? Or the piece of furniture that everyone says you should throw out, but you insist on it?

That's how you should feel about your body. You should understand that you don't need to compare it with anyone else's because it's impossible to compare unique things. In addition, who determines what beautiful and ugly mean? You should not compare your body to the celebrities' perfect-looking bodies. First, because they are adjusted with Photoshop and other programs, and they are not real. Second, because you are different, as is everybody.

CPSIA information can be obtained
at www.ICGtesting.com
Printed in the USA
BVHW041401171120
593515BV00011B/762